Curing Diseases the Chinese Way with Ginger, Garlic and Green Onion

Chief Editors

Wang Fuchun   Duan Yuhua

FOREIGN LANGUAGES PRESS   BEIJING

First Edition   1998
Second Printing   2000

Home Page:
http://www.flp.com.cn
E-mail Addresses:
Info@flp.com.cn
Sales@flp.com.cn

ISBN 7-119-01905-8

Published by Foreign Languages Press
24 Baiwanzhuang Road, Beijing 100037, China
Printed by Foreign Languages Printing House
19 Chegongzhuang Xilu, Beijing 100044, China
Distributed by China International Book Trading Corporation
35 Chegongzhuang Xilu, Beijing 100044, China
P.O. Box 399, Beijing, China
Printed in the People's Republic of China

Foreword

The Chinese people have been using green onions, ginger, and garlic as vegetables and flavoring for centuries because they are indispensable in cooking delicious food. They are also the well-known and valuable herbs used for medicinal purposes. The green onion can be used to treat rheumatic pain and numbness, abdominal pain, blood in the urine of pregnant women and breast abscesses, and can also increase lactation. The volatile allicin in garlic, as a plant bactericide, can produce a strong bactericidal effect to inhibit the growth of dysenteric bacillus and fungus of the skin and can also promote the excretion of sweat and urine, control high fever and enhance spleen functions. The volatile component in garlic can also resolve phlegm and the sulfur compound in allicin can prevent and treat hyperlipemia, improve the bodies' immune system, and prevent cancer. The volatile oil in ginger can promote blood circulation and sweating, and the gingerol in ginger can stimulate the secretion of gastric juices, promote intestinal motility, and improve digestion. The filtrate in fresh ginger can prohibit the growth of staphylococcus, vaginal trichomonad, and skin fungus.

In this book the use of green onion, ginger, and garlic in the treatment of more than one hundred medical, surgical, gynecological, pediatric, skin and ENT diseases is introduced as a simple, practical, and effective therapy. This book will be useful for home medical and also as a valuable reference for clinical practice and scientific study.

Contents

CHAPTER 1 INTRODUCTION 1
  1. Development 1
  2. Modern Investigations 5
  3. Clinical Application 8
CHAPTER 2 MEDICAL DISEASES 15
  1. Common Cold 15
  2. Cough 21
  3. Pulmonary Infection 23
  4. Asthma 24
  5. Chronic Bronchitis 26
  6. Pulmonary Tuberculosis 28
  7. Lung Abscess 31
  8. Heart Diseases 31
  9. Chest Pain 33
  10. Hypertension 34
  11. Hypotension 34
  12. Vertigo 35
  13. Hyperlipemia 35
  14. Stomachache 36
  15. Peptic Stomach Ulcer 39
  16. Hyperhydrochloria 40
  17. Chronic Gastritis 40
  18. Vomiting 40
  19. Hematemesis 43
  20. Hiccup 43
  21. Jaundice 44
  22. Hepatitis 45
  23. Cirrhosis of Liver 45
  24. Kidney Stone 45
  25. Abdominal Mass 46

26. Abdominal Distention   46
27. Abdominal Pain   47
28. Dysentery   48
29. Febrile Infectious Diseases   52
30. Cholera   53
31. Diarrhea   54
32. Indigestion   58
33. Ascites   59
34. Malaria   60
35. Constipation   61
36. Hematochezia (Anal Bleeding)   63
37. Prolapse of Anus   64
38. Cerebral Apoplexy (Stroke)   64
39. Facial Paralysis   66
40. Insomnia   67
41. Intercostal Neuralgia   67
42. Sexual Neurosis   68
43. Lumbago   68
44. Convulsion   69
45. Beriberi   69
46. Night Sweating   71
47. Leprosy   71
48. Nephritis   71
49. Dribbling Urination   72
50. Retention of Urine   73
51. Incontinence of Urine   75
52. Emission   76
53. Impotence   76
54. Bi-Syndrome (Arthritis)   76
55. Rheumatoid Arthritis   79
56. Acute Arthritis   80
57. Edema   80
58. Heat Stroke   81
59. Toxicity   82
60. Epidemic Encephalitis B   84
61. Shock   84
62. Cancer   84

63. Diabetes Mellitus 85
CHAPTER 3 SURGICAL CONDITIONS 87
  1. Boils 87
  2. Carbuncles and Cellulitis 89
  3. Erysipelas 90
  4. Tuberculosis of Cervical Lymph Nodes 90
  5. Traumatic Injuries 90
  6. Soft Tissue Injury 92
  7. Acute Sprain 93
  8. Calf Muscle Spasms 93
  9. Animal and Insect Bites 94
 10. Cut Wounds with Bleeding 94
 11. Tetanus 95
 12. Breast Ulceration 95
 13. Breast Inflammation 96
 14. Bone Fractures 97
 15. Bone Tuberculosis 97
 16. Ascaris Intestinal Obstruction 97
 17. Appendicitis 97
 18. Retention of Urine 98
 19. Difficult Urinatiion 98
 20. Scrotal Swelling and Pain 99
 21. Hernia 99
 22. Orchitis 100
 23. Swelling of Penis 101
 24. Hemorrhoids 101
 25. Pain and Swelling of Limbs 102
CHAPTER 4 GYNECOLOGICAL DISEASES 103
  1. Dysmenorrhea 103
  2. Amenorrhea 104
  3. Oligomenorrhea 105
  4. Profuse Uterine Bleeding 105
  5. Menstrual Stomachache 106
  6. Menstrual Vomiting 106
  7. Leukorrheal Disorders 106
  8. Pregnancy Vomiting 107
  9. Pregnancy Diarrhea 108

10. Pregnancy Restlessness 109
11. Habitual Abortion 109
12. Vaginal Bleeding During Pregnancy 109
13. Threatened Abortion 110
14. Retention of Lochia 110
15. Retention of Placenta 111
16. Postpartum Vomiting 111
17. Postpartum Abdominal Pain 111
18. Postpartum Edema 112
19. Postpartum Fainting 112
20. Postpartum Weakness 112
21. Oligogalactia 113
22. Breast Cancer 113
23. Hysteria 114
24. Vulvar Itching 114
25. Infertility 114
CHAPTER 5 PEDIATRIC DISEASES 116
1. Common Cold in Newborn Babies 116
2. Common Cold in Children 116
3. Bronchitis in Children 117
4. Asthma in Children 118
5. Pneumonia in Children 118
6. Whooping Cough 118
7. Chronic Cough in Children 120
8. Diarrhea in Children 120
9. Indigestion in Children 121
10. Constipation in Children 121
11. Abdominal Pain in Children 121
12. Vomiting in Children 122
13. Food Stagnation in Children 123
14. Infantile Malnutrition 124
15. Parasitic Diseases in Children 124
16. Foul Smell from Mouth in Children 126
17. Dribbling of Saliva in Children 126
18. Aphtha in Children 126
19. Incontinence of Urine in Children 127
20. Retention of Urine in Children 127

21. Epidemic Parotitis   127
22. Measles in Children   128
23. Convulsion in Children   129
24. Night Crying   129
25. Inflammation of Umbilicus in Newborn Babies   130
26. Umbilical Tetanus in Infants   130
CHAPTER 6 DERMATOLOGICAL DISEASES   131
1. Alopecia   131
2. Alopecia Areata   132
3. Grey Hair   132
4. Dandruff   132
5. Folliculitis   133
6. Eyebrow Defect   133
7. Acne Rosacea (Brandy Nose)   133
8. Tinea (Ringworm)   134
9. Psoriasis   135
10. Dermatitis   135
11. Cutaneous Pruritus   136
12. Urticaria   136
13. Eczema   136
14. Vitiligo   137
15. Tinea Versicolor   137
16. Skin Scar   137
17. Herpes Zoster   138
18. Progressive Keratosis of Finger and Palm   138
19. Desquamation of Palm   138
20. Chilblains   139
21. Wart   140
22. Underarm Odor   140
23. Clavus (Corns)   141
24. Tinea Pedis (Tinea of Foot)   142
25. Eczema of Scrotum   143
26. Impetigo   143
27. Chronic Ulceration in Perineal Region   143
CHAPTER 7 DISEASES OF EAR, NOSE AND THROAT   145
1. Rhinitis   145
2. Nasal Bleeding   146

3. Toothache   146
4. Periodontitis   147
5. Aphtha of Mouth Cavity   148
6. Sore Throat   148
7. Laryngitis   149
8. Diphtheria   149
9. Aphonia   150
10. Hoarseness of Voice   150
11. Foreign Body in Throat   151
12. Conjunctivitis   151
13. Itching of Eye   152
14. Profuse Lacrimation   152
15. Deafness   152
16. Otitis Media   153
17. Insect in Ear   153

Chapter 1
INTRODUCTION

1. Development

Green onion, ginger, and garlic have pungent odors and warm natures and are capable of expelling cold and improving the appetite. In daily life they are indispensable flavorings for cooking delicious food. At the same time, they are valuable herbs with an important role in the prevention and treatment of diseases, used for thousands of years.

As early as the Eastern Han Dynasty (A.D.25-220), the green onion had been used by physicians as a common herb to treat many conditions. As mentioned in the *Shen Nong's Materia Medica*, the earliest extant medical treatise, white stalk of green onion is indicated for febrile infectious disease with chills, fever, sweating, and edema of the face and eyes. The adoption of this herb for medical use began in very ancient time because it was a plant easy to grow and widely distributed in China. As a herb, it has been mentioned in many medical and herbal books since *Shen Nong's Materia Medica* was written. In the *Informal Records of Famous Physicians* written centuries ago, we read that it can be used to treat headaches due to febrile infectious diseases. During the Ming Dynasty (1368-1644), Li Shizhen, the great medical scholar, widely expanded the clinical application of green onion by incorporating the experiences of medical specialists in previous dynasties and accumulating his own knowledge after clinical practice and observation. In the Yuan and Ming dynasties (1271-1644), the white stalk of green onion was used for many medical, surgical, gynecological and pediatric diseases. By the Qing Dynasty (1644-1911), the functions of different parts of the green onion had been clearly distinguished. As stated in the *New Compilation of Materia Medica* written by Wu Yiluo, the green onion is used to promote sweating and the circulation of qi (vital energy). It is also used to remove stagnation in blood vessels and restore yang, especially in patients with a flushed face, vomiting, and retention of urine and stool. He also pointed out the differences between the white stalk and green leaf: "The white stalk has a pungent odor and a warm nature; the green leaf also has a pungent taste, but a cold nature." Therefore they are used to treat different diseases. After the extensive application of green onion in clinical practice over a long period of time, physicians found it to be incompatible with honey in the same prescription, but a mixture of these two herbs is an effective preparation for infection of the gums.

Ginger is widely grown in China and various parts and different preparations of ginger may produce different therapeutic effects. The juice squeezed from the fresh root is called ginger juice, and the root skin is called ginger peel. The roasted ginger is a herb prepared by roasting over fire, but dried ginger is prepared by direct airing. Ginger was first mentioned in *Informal Records of Famous Physicians* as an important herb useful for treating febrile infectious diseases with headache, nasal obstruction, coughing and shortness of breath and to stop vomiting. Since then, ginger has been widely used and discussed by many medical books. For example, in *A Supplement to the Herbal* written by Chen Cangqi of the Tang Dynasty (618-907), ginger juice was claimed useful for relieving the toxic effect of drugs and improving appetite. Therefore, ginger is often used to relieve the toxic effects of *banxia* (半 夏 , Ternate Pinellia), *nanxing* (南 星 , Rhizoma Arisaematis), fish and crab poisoning and to control vomiting. In the Ming Dynasty, Li Shizhen summarized the use of fresh ginger and roasted ginger: "The fresh ginger is used for expelling pathogenic factors and the roasted ginger for adjusting the spleen and stomach." Later, roasted ginger was recommended for the treatment of hemorrhage and dried ginger for syndromes of the spleen and stomach caused by cold. Dried ginger is the dry root of ginger. As mentioned in the *Shen Nong's Materia Medica* it is used to relieve fullness in the chest, coughing, and shortness of breath, and to warm the spleen and stomach, stop bleeding and promote sweating, treat rheumatic arthritis, and control dysentery and diarrhea. In another medical book the four functions of dried ginger are listed as promoting and supporting heart yang, removing cold in internal organs, expelling cold qi from meridians, and treating abdominal pain caused by cold. The ginger peel has a pungent odor and a cool nature and can produce a strong diuretic effect. The ginger peel is usually prescribed with *fulingpi* (茯 苓 皮 , Poria peel), *sangbaipi* (桑 白 皮 , Root Bark of White Mulberry) and *dafupi* (大 腹 皮 , Shell of Areca Nut) to compound the prescription *wupi yin* (Decoction of Peel of Five Herbs) for inducing diuresis and resolving edema. Zhang Zhongjing, a medical sage of the Eastern Han Dynasty (25-220), created many prescriptions containing ginger, such as *xiaoqinglong tang* (Minor Decoction of Green Dragon), *guizhi tang* (Cinnamon Twig Decoction), *sanwu beiji tang* (Decoction of Three Herbs for Emergency), *xiaochaihu tang* (Minor Decoction of Root of Chinese Thorowax), *dachaihu tang* (Major Decoction of Root of Chinese Thorowax), and *banxia xiexin tang* (Decoction of Pinellia for Purging Stomach Fire). These demonstrated the important medical value of ginger in clinical practice.

Garlic is a perennial lily bulb, easily grown everywhere in China and used over thousands of years as an important herb by common people for treating parasites, toxicity, edema and swelling, and blood stasis. As a formal herb, garlic was first mentioned in the *Commentaries on Shen Nong's Materia Medica*, written by Tao Hongjing (456-536). It has a pungent odor, warm nature, and wide indications. As mentioned in the *Informal*

Records of Famous Physicians, the garlic can treat pyogenic infection, expel wind pathogen and relieve toxicity. In the *Tang Materia Medica* by Su Jing, the functions of garlic for transporting qi downward and promoting digestion of grains and meat are mentioned. It was also used externally for sterilization and for garlic moxibustion at that time. A garlic slice with pin holes is put on the acupoint or swollen lesions for moxibustion with moxa cones for the treatment of tuberculosis of the lymph nodes. In the *Essence of Surgery*, written by Chen Ziming in the Ming Dynasty, garlic is mentioned for the treatment of carbuncles at their early stage. In the collection of *Dietetic Materia Medica* written by Shen Jilong of the Qing Dynasty, the paste of garlic mixed with sesame oil is externally applied to treat various pyogenic infections. In a book written by Wang Shixiong of the Qing Dynasty, the uses of garlic were summarized. Fresh garlic is pungent and hot, cooked garlic sweet and warm. Garlic can be used to remove the cold and damp of yin pathogens, transport qi downward, warm the spleen and stomach, promote the digestion of grains and meat, release accumulated cold, treat acute abdominal pain and diarrhea, relieve retention of urine and stool, treat toxicity of dirty pathogens, relieve abdominal distention, kill parasites, promote the discharge of water, and stop nasal bleeding. Moxibustion with garlic can cure carbuncles and cellulitis. After putting the patient in a prone posture, 500 mg of garlic paste is applied to the back from Dazhui (GV 14) to Yaoshu (GV 2) and moxibustion is applied over the garlic paste until the smell of garlic can be detected, then the garlic paste is removed with warm water. Garlic paste mixed with a small amount of plant oil is applied around the anus before going to bed to prevent and treat hookworm and pinworm infection. In recent years, the uses of garlic have been markedly increased with about a hundred kinds of diseases now curable by this herb, including pulmonary tuberculosis, whooping cough, dysentery, diarrhea, influenza, appendicitis, and hypertension.

In the medical history of China, the green onion, ginger and garlic were used extensively from very ancient time among common people as effective drugs and delicious flavoring, and both uses are valuable to health.

2. Modern Investigations

To study the therapeutic mechanisms of the green onion, ginger and garlic, Chinese medical professionals have carried on wide-ranging scientific investigations.

1. Green onion

1) Scientific name, distribution, and function: The green onion (Herba Allium Fistulosum L.) can be grown everywhere in China and is harvested through the warm seasons with the fresh stalk and leaf used for medical and cooking purposes. This plant has a pungent odor and warm nature producing therapeutic effects through the lung and stomach meridians and can induce sweating, expel cold, activate yang, relieve toxicity, and remove stagnation.

2) Composition: This plant contains onion oil, malic acid, Vitamins B and C and iron salt.

3) Pharmacological effects: The green onion can induce sweating to reduce fever, strengthen the stomach and promote the discharge of urine and phlegm, because the onion oil excreted from the lungs can stimulate the secretion of bronchi to produce an expectorant effect.

2. Ginger

1) Scientific name, distribution and function: The fresh ginger (Rhizoma Zingiberis Recens) is the root of the Zingiberaceae, a perennial plant, grown all over the country and harvested in autumn (from Sept. to Nov.). The herb is prepared and stored for use after removing the fine roots. Washed and cut into slices it has a pungent odor and a warm nature to produce therapeutic effects through the spleen and lung meridians. Fresh ginger can induce sweating, and stop vomiting by warm-

ing the spleen and stomach and can control coughing by warming the lungs.

Dried ginger is prepared by drying fresh ginger harvested in the winter in sunshine or in an oven and then cut into slices for use. This herb has a pungent odor and a hot nature producing therapeutic effects through the spleen, stomach, heart, and lung meridians. It can be used to warm the spleen, stomach, and lungs, restore yang, and remove excessive fluid retained in the body.

Roasted ginger is prepared by baking fresh ginger until the surface turns light black and the interior turns brown in color. This herb has a bitter and astringent taste and a warm nature producing therapeutic effects through the liver and spleen meridians. It is used to warm the meridians and stop bleeding, but its effectiveness in warming the internal organs is weaker than that of dried ginger.

Ginger peel is the skin cut from fresh ginger. It has a pungent odor and cool nature to strengthen the spleen and promote the discharge of fluid from the body.

2) Composition: The chief chemical components of ginger are zingiberol, zingiberene, phellandrene, camphene, citral, and linalool. After decomposition, the gingerol (a chemical component with a pungent odor) may form a mixture of shogoal (an oily pungent element) and zingiberone (a crystal pungent element).

3) Pharmacological effects: The volatile oil of ginger can promote peripheral blood circulation to induce sweating and produce a warm sensation in the body, stimulate the secretion of gastric juices and motility of the stomach and intestine, improve appetite, inhibit abnormal fermentation in the intestines, promote the discharge of intestinal gas, adjust and improve the functions of the stomach, and control vomiting. As demonstrated in laboratory experiments, ginger can also produce an anti-inflammatory and analgesic effect.

3. Garlic

1) Scientific name, distribution and function: Garlic (Bulbus

Allium Sativum) is the bulb of the lily family, a perennial herbaceous plant, grown all over China and harvested in May after the leaves have withered. Dried garlic used as a herb has a pungent odor and a warm nature producing a therapeutic effect through the lungs, spleen, and stomach meridians, and resolving edema and swelling, relieving toxicity, killing parasites, expelling phlegm, and increasing the discharge of urine.

2) Composition: Allicin is an important component with an antibiotic effect, accounting for 1.5 percent of the plant. It is a yellow liquid material with a strong foul odor, destroyed by heat and alkali, but not by diluted acid. In recent years, a new bactericidal component, neoallicin (diallyl thiosul fonate), has been discovered by Chinese pharmacologists.

3) Pharmacological effects:

(1) Antibiotic effect: The volatile oil of garlic may produce a strong bactericidal effect. In a 0.5 percent water solution it can kill typhoid bacillus within 5 minutes. Garlic juice, garlic extract and allicin all have apparent bacteriostatic and bactericidal effects on staphylococcus, meningococcus, diphtheria bacillus, dysentery bacillus, Bacillus coli, typhoid bacillus, paratyphoid bacillus, tuberculous bacillus, and Vibriochlerae. The therapeutic effect of purple skin garlic is better than that of white skin garlic. The phytocidin, a garlic preparation, is sensitive to bacteria with resistance to penicillin, streptomycin, chloromycetin, and aureomycin. In a liquid medium, garlic may inhibit the growth of tuberculous bacillus, but the bacteriostatic effect can be reduced in the presence of serum.

(2) Antiprotozoal and antitrichomonal effect: Amebae lose activity after contact with a 5-15 percent solution of garlic. As proved by experiments with direct contact or double a distilling method, garlic juice may kill all Trichomonas in test tubes within 15-25 minutes, and the volatile component may kill them within 90-180 minutes. The 0.5 percent garlic filtrate may inhibit the motility of Trichomonas vaginalis within 5 minutes.

(3) Enhancement of digestion: The oral ingestion of garlic

may improve appetite and promote secretions of the stomach and the motility of stomach and intestines through direct stimulation and reflex reaction.

(4) Effect on cardiovascular system: According to clinical observation of 114 cases of hypertension and atherosclerosis, garlic markedly reduced systolic blood pressure by 1.1-4.4 kPa, and diastolic pressure by 0.5 to 2.7 kPa, and this hypotensive effect could not be blocked by bilateral vagotomy or by injection of atropine.

(5) Inhibition of aggregation of blood platelets: The oral administration of garlic oil or garlic itself may inhibit the aggregation of platelets caused by ADP and adrenalin. The oral intake of garlic over a long period of time may prevent arteriosclerosis.

(6) Garlic can also produce apparent anti-inflammatory, anti-tumorous, hypoglycemic, and lipid-reducing effects.

3. Clinical Application

1. Application of green onion

1) The green onion is often used in combination with ginger and *dandouchi* (淡 豆 豉, medicated soybean) to induce sweating and relieve external syndromes in patients with mild influenza of the wind-cold type. It may be combined with ginger to compound a prescription called *lianxu congbai tang* (Decoction with Ginger and Stalk of Green Onion), or combined with *dandouchi* to form *congchi tang* (Decoction with Green Onion and Medicated Soybean Decoction).

2) The green onion can be used to treat excessive cold yin pathogen in the body. It is combined with *fuzi* (附 子, Aconite), and dried ginger to compose a prescription called *baitong tang* (Decoction for Activating Yang and Dispelling Cold) to treat diarrhea, cold limbs, and weak pulse; and hot fried green onion may be used as a hot compress over the abdomen around umbilicus to treat cold pain in the abdomen due to stagnation of qi and accumulation of cold, and to treat retention of urine

due to functional imapirment of the urinary bladder.

3) The external application of green onion paste may treat ulcers, carbuncles and furuncles; and a mixture with honey may produce a good therapeutic effect in treating toxicity and stagnation, but the mixture with honey should not be orally administered.

2. Application of ginger

1) Fresh ginger:

(1) A hot decoction of fresh ginger and brown sugar can be administered to treat mild influenza with chills, fever, and nasal obstruction due to an attack of external wind and cold pathogens.

(2) Fresh ginger may be combined with *banxia* (半 夏, Ternate Pinellia) to compose a prescription called *xiaobanxia tang* (Minor Decoction of Ternate Pinellia) to treat vomiting due to cold in the stomach; and it may be combined with *zhuru* (竹 茹, Caudis Bambosae in Taenia) and *huanglian* (黄 连, Goldthread) to treat vomiting with heat in the stomach.

(3) It may be used to treat cough due to an attack of wind and cold pathogens.

(4) It also may be used to treat toxicity of *banxia* (半 夏, Ternate Pinellia), *nanxing* (南 星, Rhizoma Arisaematis), fish and turtle. It can not be used in patients with internal deficiency and excessive heat.

(5) It may be used to treat rheumatic arthralgia and lumbago. A 5-10 percent solution of fresh ginger was injected to tender spots, tender nodules, and local and remote acupoints in 113 patients with rheumatic arthralgia and chronic lumbago. In effective cases, the pain was reduced or relieved, the swelling of joints was resolved or improved, and the locomotive function was recovered or improved after treatment.

(6) It also may be used to treat gastric and duodenal ulcers. Fifty gram of fresh ginger was boiled in 300 ml of water for 30 minutes after being washed clean and cut into small pieces, and was administered to ten-odd patients, 3 times a day for 2 days.

After treatment, pain was reduced or relieved, appetite was improved, and constipation and black stool was relieved, but the obstruction sensation was retained in some patients over a long time and the symptoms recurred.

(7) It may be used to treat acute dysentery. In 50 dysenteric patients, abdominal and rectal pain was relieved 5-16 days and 5-14 days respectively after treatment with fresh ginger paste.

(8) It may be used to treat intestinal obstruction caused by roundworm. Among 109 patients treated with a mixture of ginger and honey, 104 cases were cured.

2) Dried ginger:

(1) Dried ginger is used to treat cold symdrome of the spleen and stomach accompanied by cold and pain in the abdomen, vomiting, and diarrhea. It may be prescribed with *renshen* (人参, Ginseng), *baizhu* (白 术, Largehead Atractylodis) and *gancao* (甘 草, Licorice) to compose a prescription called *lizhong wan* (Pill for Regulating Spleen and Stomach) for treatment of cold deficient syndrome of the spleen and stomach.

(2) It may be used with *fuzi* (附 子, Aconite) to treat yang depletion syndrome by promoting the circulation of heart yang, enriching yang and expelling internal cold.

(3) It may be used with *mahuang* (麻 黄, Herba Ephedra), *xixin* (细 辛, Wildginger) and *wuweizi* (五 味 子, Chinese Magnoliavine) to treat cold in the body and back, cough and asthma with profuse thin phlegm due to accumulation of cold fluid in the lungs.

Dried ginger should be carefully prescribed to pregnant women.

3) Roasted ginger: It is used to treat bleeding diseases such as spitting blood, blood in stool, and profuse uterine bleeding in patients with a pale complexion, cold limbs, pale tongue, and thready pulse.

4) Ginger peel: It is used with *fulingpi* (茯 苓 皮, Poria peel), *sangbaipi* (桑 白 皮, Root Bark of White Mulberry), *dafupi* (大 腹 皮, Shell of Areca Nut) and *jupi* (橘 皮, dried

tangerine peel) to treat edema.

3. Application of garlic

1) Garlic can be used to treat tinea and pyogenic infections, such as carbuncles and furuncles. The application of a thick layer of an oily paste of garlic can resolve swelling. Tinea of the scalp can be cured by rubbing with garlic slices or an application of garlic paste.

2) It may be used to treat pulmonary tuberculosis, whooping cough, dysentery, and diarrhea. Garlic with purple skin in the amount of 30 g is boiled in water for 1-1.5 minutes, and after the garlic is removed, 30 g of rice is boiled in the garlic water to cook a rice soup. The rice soup, together with the boiled garlic and 3 g of *baiji* (白 芨, Bletilla) powder, is taken twice a day for 3 months to treat pulmonary tuberculosis. Thirty grams of the paste of garlic with purple skin is soaked in 60 g of cool boiled water for 12 hours, and one spoonful of this garlic extract is administered three times a day for 10-15 days. For treatment of dysentery and diarrhea, fresh garlic or a decoction of garlic may be taken orally, and 100 ml of 10 percent garlic extract may be used for a retention enema once a day for one week.

3) It may be used to prevent and treat influenza and to treat crab toxicity.

Cautions: Because of the stimulant nature of garlic, it can not be used to treat patients with diseases of the eyes, teeth, throat and tongue due to deficiency of yin and excessive fire; the external application of garlic should not be retained for a long time, because it may cause redness, heat, and skin blisters, and the garlic solution retention enema is prohibited for use with pregnant women.

4) It may be used to treat bacillary dysentery. An apparent effectiveness was obtained in 43 cases among 65 dysentery patients treated with allicin. The effective rate was 67.8 percent in dysenteric patients treated with 12 percent garlic solution by oral administration or retention enema. Treatment was contin-

ued for 2 weeks after the symptoms were relieved.

5) It may be used to treat amebic dysentery. In 100 patients with amebic dysentery, one bulb of garlic was orally administered daily for one week, and an enema with a 10 percent garlic solution was given once a day for one week. The rate of cure with this treatment was 88 percent. The patients were treated with an oral administration of 1-3 bulbs of garlic or retention enema with 5 percent water extract of garlic per day for 5-10 days.

6) It may be used to treat fungus infection. An injection of garlic solution may produce certain therapeutic effects in treating fungus infection of the lungs and digestive system, and cryptococcus meningitis. The total effective rate in 16 cases of cryptococcus meningitis treated with an intravenous drip infusion of garlic solution in a 10 percent glucose solution was 68.8 percent. The effective rate reached 93 percent in fungus infections of the lungs and digestive system, and the therapeutic effect was also satisfactory for fungal vaginitis.

7) It may be used to treat whooping cough. The therapeutic effect of a 10-20 percent garlic extract was satisfactory in the treatment of whooping cough and whooping cough with pneumonia. Among 100 cases of whooping cough treated with allicin, 54 cases were cured.

8) It may be used to treat tuberculosis of the trachea. Among cases with tuberculosis of the trachea treated with an intravenous drip infusion of 1-5 percent garlic solution, 31 cases were cured after a short follow-up team, one case was improved, and one case remained unchanged.

9) It may be used to treat acute appendicitis. The therapeutic effective rate was above 90 percent in patients with acute appendicitis treated by external applications of garlic paste or a paste of garlic and mirabilite. An effective rate of 81 percent was obtained in patients treated with a garlic solution.

10) The application of **garlic paste** with small amounts of plant oil around the anus may quickly kill newly hatched

pinworms.

11) It may be used to treat trichomoniasis. A gelatin-glycerol suppository of 50 percent garlic or sitz bath with 5-10 percent garlic solution for 7-10 days may be used to treat vaginal trichomoniasis. An enema with 100ml of 100 percent garlic extract, 1-2 times a day, and atabrine 0.1 g twice a day may be used to treat intestinal trichomoniasis. Symptoms may improve 3 days after treatment, with complete recovery 5-7 day after treatment.

12) It may be used to treat hyperlipemia. The triglyceride and cholesterol blood levels may be reduced in patients with hyperlipemia after treatment with capsules of garlic oil.

13) It may be used to treat tumors. The nasopharyngeal squamous cell carcinoma, lympho-epithelioma, undifferentiated small cell carcinoma of the lungs, squamous cell carcinoma of cardia and adenocarcinoma of the stomach are sensitive to treatment with injections of garlic solution. After 10-15 days of treatment with an intravenous drip infusion of garlic solution, the cervical masses in a large number of patients with nasopharyngeal carcinoma were reduced in size and symptoms improved or relieved.

14) It can be used to prevent lead poisoning. After treatment of lead poisoning with garlic slices (0.3 g per slice), 4 pieces twice a day for one month, symptoms in the digestive system were apparently improved, the purine determination of urine turned negative in 85 percent of patients, and the delta-ALA in urine was reduced to normal levels in all patients.

15) It can be used to treat epidemic meningitis and encephalitis B. After treatment with an intramuscular injection of 10 percent distillate of garlic (diluted with 0.5 percent procaine), 84 cases of ordinary epidemic meningitis were all cured. The oral administration of garlic may prevent epidemic meningitis and the drip infusion of a garlic solution may produce good therapeutic results in treating of encephalitis B.

16) It can be used to treat hypertension. After a treatment

with garlic for 3-5 days in 100 cases of hypertension, vertigo, headache, and backache all disappeared and blood pressure was reduced by more than 2.7 kPa in 40 percent of the patients.

17) It may be used to treat clavus. The surrounding skin of the clavus is protected with adhesive plaster and garlic paste with small amounts of white stalk of green onion is applied over the clavus. A few days later, the clavus may turn black and shed off.

18) It may be used to treat pyogenic surgical infection. A 10 percent garlic solution is prepared with 10 ml of garlic juice, 90 ml of normal saline and 1 ml of 0.5 percent procaine and the gauze soaked with this solution is used to fill or cover the infected lesions, while the dressing is changed once a day. New granulation tissue may appear and grow 3-5 days later, and the wound may heal 5-7 days after that.

Although the toxicity of garlic and its preparation is very low, it may produce a strong stimulation to the local tissues when applied externally. Garlic should be carefully prescribed to patients with kidney diseases, because it is irritating to the kidneys parenchyma.

Chapter 2
MEDICAL DISEASES

1. Common Cold

Recipe 1: Fresh ginger 15 g, green onion stalk 15 g, and pear 120 g.

Prescription: Above three ingredients are boiled in water and poured into a bowl with two beaten eggs. The patient should lie in bed covered with a heavy blanket to induce sweating after drinking this hot decoction.

Explanation: The stalk of green onion and ginger have a pungent odor and warm nature to expel cold pathogen and relieve exterior syndromes; the pear can increase body fluid and clear heat in the lungs; and the egg can nourish yin and moisten dryness in the body. As a drug to relieve exterior syndromes and regulate lung functions, this decoction can be used to treat common cold caused by an attack of wind and cold pathogens on the body surface and a disturbance of lung functions. It is especially useful for curing coughs.

Recipe 2: Garlic 15 g and vinegar 15 ml.

Prescription: A garlic paste is mixed with vinegar to prepare a sauce for a meal of noodles (or rice noodles). The patient should lie in bed to induce sweating after taking the noodles with a garlic and vinegar sauce.

Explanation: The garlic and vinegar can clear up heat and toxic pathogens. This preparation is very effective for curing the common cold and for preventing influenza.

Recipe 3: Fresh ginger 3-5 g, 5-7 green onion stalks with fine roots, glutinous rice 50-100 g and vinegar 10-15 ml.

Prescription: The glutinous rice and ginger are boiled in water in an earthenware pot for 1 minute and then boiled with stalks of green onion to prepare a rice soup. After mixing with vinegar and slightly boiled for a while, the hot rice soup, or just the liquid portion of the soup, may be taken. Afterward, the patient should have a nap under a thick blanket to induce slight sweating.

Explanation: It is said that when Emperor Wenzong of the Yuan Dynasty was on an inspection tour in the south he caught a cold. After eating this porridge he was in high spirits. Hence the name of "immortal porridge."

Recipe 4: An adequate amount of garlic.

Prescription: After the garlic is juiced, the garlic juice is diluted with ten times the amount of water for application as nose drops. As an alternative, 2 pieces of garlic may be kept in the mouth for continuous sucking.

Explanation: This is a convenient method for preventing the common cold. Right after the appearance of symptoms such as chills, adequate preventive procedures should be adopted.

Recipe 5: An adequate amount of fresh ginger and brown sugar.

Prescription: The fresh ginger and brown sugar are boiled and drunk to induce sweating after taking a nap under a thick blanket.

Explanation: This is another convenient method for preventing the common cold. The brown sugar can promote blood circulation and the ginger can induce sweating by its hot nature.

Recipe 6: Garlic and ginger.

Prescription: The garlic juice or the hot water extract of small bits of garlic and ginger may be drunk to induce sweating. The chopped garlic and ginger may be added to a sauce for a meal of noodles.

Explanation: This is a method of treating patients in the

early stages of the common cold without sweating, namely, in a stage of exterior syndrome. Both garlic and ginger have a pungent odor and a warm nature, therefore, they can expel cold pathogen and relieve exterior syndrome.

Recipe 7: Six green onion stalks, dried ginger 30 g and *dandouchi* (淡 豆 豉, Medicated Soybean) 12 g.

Prescription: The sliced ginger, sliced and pounded stalk of green onion, and *douchi* are boiled in a cup of water until half a cup of decoction is obtained. The hot decoction with the dregs removed may be drunk to induce sweating by wearing a heavy overcoat or having a nap under a heavy blanket.

Explanation: This is a recipe used only at the early stages of the common cold with nasal obstruction and headache, but without sweating, because all three ingredients warm the body and induce sweating.

Recipe 8: Green onion stalks, 7-8 pieces, and a small handful of *dandouchi* (淡 豆 豉, Medicated Soybean).

Prescription: The pounded stalks of green onion and *douchi* are boiled in water and a cup of decoction is drunk to induce sweating and expel wind pathogen after having a nap under a heavy blanket. Then the patient may feel relaxed and comfortable.

Explanation: This is a recipe to treat the common cold in the early stages with cold pathogen invading only the body surface.

Recipe 9: Green onion stalks 25 g, and ginger 25 g.

Prescription: A warm water decoction of green onion and ginger is orally administered.

Explanation: This is a method for treating the common cold in the early stages when the patient should avoid a further attack of wind pathogen.

Recipe 10: Three bulbs of garlic and 10 pieces of green onion stalks.

Prescription: The chopped garlic and green onion are put into a rice soup, and after further boiling for a short time, the hot rice soup may be taken by the patients and their body warmth should be maintained by wearing a heavy overcoat or having a nap under a heavy blanket.

Explanation: This is a method for treating the common cold in the early stages, especially useful for patients with headache.

Recipe 11: Green onion stalks 15 g, ginger 15 g, and tea leaves 9 g.

Prescription: The chopped green onion and sliced ginger are boiled with the tea leaves in a pot with one and a half cups of water, and the hot decoction is taken after the dregs are removed.

Explanation: The tea leaf is an effective ingredient for relieving headache. Therefore, it is often included in the recipes of patent herbal drugs for the common cold. Through the course of treatment, the patient should avoid further attacks by wind.

Recipe 12: Fresh ginger 50 g, brown sugar 50 g, and tea leaves 2.5 g.

Prescription: The water decoction of these three ingredients is administered to the patient. He should then take a nap after eating a hot rice soup.

Explanation: This is a method used to treat the common cold in its early stages with severe headache, because the three ingredients can strengthen the spleen and stomach to expel cold from body.

Recipe 13: Fresh ginger 6-7 slices and *dandouchi* (淡 豆 豉 , Medicated Soybean) 20 g.

Prescription: Boil these three ingredients and the hot decoction is taken by the patient. Then the patient should take a nap under a heavy blanket.

Explanation: The fresh ginger can expel cold pathogen, and *dandouchi* can relieve symptoms of the common cold. In combination they can effectively relieve headache in the early stage of a cold.

Recipe 14: Fresh ginger 50 g, some brown sugar, and a stalk of green onion.

Prescription: The chopped fresh ginger, brown sugar, and stalk of green onion are soaked in boiled water or boiled in water for a while to prepare an instant hot drink for inducing sweating. The patient should drink it while it is hot, and take a nap under a heavy blanket.

Explanation: This is a method for treating the common cold with cold and abdominal pain caused by drenching rain.

Recipe 15: One piece of green onion stalk.

Prescription: Cut the stalk of green onion and put it just beneath the nostrils, or paste a slice of sticky layer of the white bulb of green onion on the upper lip under the nostrils. The patient is asked to take deep breaths until the nasal obstruction is relieved.

Explanation: This is a method for treating nasal obstruction, which can be relieved by the irritable odor of green onion.

Recipe 16: One piece of green onion and a spoonful of red chili oil.

Prescription: In the early stages of the common cold, thin hot noodle soup cooked with green onion and a spoonful of red chili oil may be taken to expel pathogens.

Explanation: This is a method to relieve nasal obstruction of the common cold after the wind and cold pathogens are expelled.

Recipe 17: Green onion stalks, 6-7 pieces, and an adequate amount of ginger slices and pepper.

Prescription: The fine bits of green onion are fried in plant oil, then added to a noodles with some boiled water. If some ginger slices and pepper powder are added to the noodles at the same time, the therapeutic effect may be even better.

Explanation: After frying, the stalk of green onion may produce a better effect for expelling external pathogens. After adding ginger slices and pepper powder, the noodles can stimulate the excretion of nasal discharge and sweat, produce a warm sensation in the body, and effectively relieve nasal obstruction.

Recipe 18: An adequate amount of garlic, ginger slices, green onion, and pepper powder.

Prescription: A meal of wheat flour flakes is cooked by boiling in water with garlic, ginger slices, and green onion. Right before the meal is taken, some pepper powder may be added and the running nose can be controlled after the meal.

Explanation: This method is useful for treating nasal obstruction in patients with a common cold. During the course of treatment they should avoid further exposure to wind.

Recipe 19: Three slices of ginger, one piece of dried root of Chinese cabbage, and brown sugar 50 g.

Prescription: A hot decoction is made by boiling the above three ingredients in the water. The patient takes three times a day.

Explanation: This method is used to treat the common cold due to an attack of wind and cold pathogens by clearing up heat, inducing urination, and expelling pathogens from the body surface.

Recipe 20: Fresh ginger slices 25 g, meat of a carp fish 150 g, and rice wine 100 ml.

Prescription: The sliced fish meat, ginger slices, and rice wine are put into a bowl with half a bowl of boiled water and steamed for thirty minutes. After adding some salt and flavorings, the hot steamed fish may be taken to slightly induce sweating when the patient lies in bed covered with a heavy blanket. The steamed fish may be taken twice a day and the patients should avoid further attacks of wind and cold pathogens.

Explanation: This method can be used to expel wind and cold pathogens from the body surface and control pain in patients with a common cold with chills, headache, fatigue and nasal obstruction.

Recipe 21: Four pieces of green onion stalks, egg white of 2 duck eggs, and malt sugar 50 g.

Prescription: The green onion stalks and malt sugar are boiled in two cups of water for a few minutes, and then poured into a bowl with the duck egg whites to prepare a soup by stirring them well. The soup is then eaten, one half at a time, during the course of one day. The patient should avoid sour and spicy food.

Explanation: This method is used to nourish yin and clear up heat in patients with a common cold including coughing, hoarseness, and sore and swollen throat.

2. Cough

Recipe 1: One piece of green onion and one duck egg.

Prescription: The chopped green onion and the fresh duck egg are mixed in a bowl with boiled water. After taking the hot soup, the patient should lie in bed under a heavy blanket and the cough may be cured after a short nap.

Explanation: This is a method used to treat coughs in patients with a common cold.

Recipe 2: Half a spoonful of ginger juice and one spoonful of malt sugar.

Prescription: The ginger juice and malt sugar are mixed in boiled water for administration 2-3 times a day.

Explanation: This is an inexpensive treatment for chronic coughs in aged people.

Recipe 3: Fresh ginger 10 g, fresh leaf mustard 80 g, and a small amount of table salt.

Prescription: After washing clean, the leaf mustard is cut into small pieces and the ginger into slices. They are then boiled in four bowls of water until two bowls of decoction is obtained, adding some salt. Take it one bowl each time, twice a day. A good therapeutic result may be obtained after treatment for three days.

Explanation: This recipe is used to treat cough, headache, and aching pains in the limbs caused by wind and cold pathogens.

Recipe 4: Six pieces of green onion stalks, fresh ginger 15 g, and one radish.

Prescription: The radish is well boiled in three bowls of water and then is continuously boiled after the stalk of green onion and ginger are added, until one bowl of soup is obtained for one administration with its solid contents.

Explanation: This preparation can improve ventilation of the lungs, relieve exterior syndrome, resolve phlegm, and control cough to treat patient with coughing, foamy sputum, chills, fatigue, and soreness and pains in the body.

Recipe 5: Fresh ginger 15 g, date 30 g, and brown sugar 30 g.

Prescription: The three ingredients are boiled in three bowls of water and the decoction is taken to induce slight sweating.

Explanation: This method can expel wind and cold pathogens when treating patients with a common cold including cough, coldness, pricking pains in the stomach, and postpartum diarrhea due to an attack of cold pathogen and pregnant hyperemesis.

Recipe 6: Fresh ginger three slices, one radish, five pieces of white pepper and one piece of *chenpi* (陈 皮, Dried Tangerine Peel).

Prescription: The ingredients are boiled in water for 30 minutes. It is eaten twice a day.

Explanation: This method can check an adverse ascending of qi and resolve phlegm to treat coughing with profuse sputum.

Recipe 7: An adequate amount of fresh ginger, cane sugar 50 g, and one egg.

Prescription: The half-bowl boiled sugar solution is mixed with the beaten egg and ginger juice for one drink, twice a day.

Explanation: This method can treat chronic cough due to a

deficiency of essence in the body.

Recipe 8: Fresh ginger 5 g, brown sugar 10 g and walnuts 10 g.

Prescription: The sugar is melted in a metal soup ladle over a slow fire and then baked with ginger and walnuts until they turn dark brown. The baked preparation is taken 1-2 times a day for several days after the ginger is removed.

Explanation: This method can treat cough due to an attack of wind and cold pathogens, because the fresh ginger can expel wind and cold pathogens.

Recipe 9: Fresh ginger juice, pear juice, and white radish juice 30 g of each.

Prescription: The egg white is beaten well with the mixed juice for administration.

Explanation: This method is used to treat chronic cough.

Recipe 10: Garlic 500 g and an adequate amount of cane sugar.

Prescription: Pound the garlic into paste. Two spoonfuls of garlic paste mixed with sugar is taken with hot water twice a day.

Explanation: This method is used to treat cough caused by an attack of wind and cold pathogens.

3. Pulmonary Infection

Recipe 1: Garlic with purple skin 60 g and vinegar 100 ml.

Prescription: The garlic and vinegar are boiled in an earthenware pot for 10-15 minutes as a drink after meals. Twice a day over a long period of time.

Explanation: This preparation should be taken after meals to reduce irritative discomfort in the stomach and intestines.

Recipe 2: 10 percent garlic solution 20 ml.

Prescription: Spray inhalation of this solution, twice a day.

Explanation: Fungal infection of the lungs is usually caused by Candida albicans and the patients may suffer from low fever, weakness, and coughing with mucoid or bloody sputum. If fungal pneumonia develops, the patients may have high fever and exacerbated symptoms. An X-ray of the chest may show peribronchitis or bronchopneumonia. This disease may take a chronic course and the patient may develop mycotic stomatitis as a complication.

4. Asthma

Recipe 1: *Dilong* (地 龙, Earthworm) 30 g and fresh ginger 30 g.

Prescription: They are boiled to prepare a decoction for administration two times a day for 5-7 days.

Explanation: This is a recipe to treat bronchial asthma, and the patient is prohibited from smoking, drinking alcohol, and eating uncooked, cold, greasy or fishy food.

Recipe 2: Garlic 30 g

Prescription: Pound garlic into paste and then put the paste over the Yongquan (KI 1) acupoints in the bilateral soles and wrapped in gauze. The garlic is changed every day for several days or until the attack is controlled.

Explanation: This method is used to treat cough and asthma with profuse or bloody sputum. The patient should keep his feet warm and is prohibited from smoking, drinking alcohol, and eating spicy food.

Recipe 3: Fresh ginger juice 150 g and brown sugar 120 g.

Prescription: The ingredients are boiled in water for 20 minutes and half a spoonful of decoction is slowly swallowed.

Explanation: This recipe can be used to resolve phlegm, check the adverse ascent of qi, warm the spleen and stomach, control asthma, and treat asthma with sputum in aged people.

Recipe 4: Fresh ginger juice 3 ml, juice of white radish 200 ml, and honey 30 ml.

Prescription: The mixed juice is drunk once a day after being slightly boiled.

Explanation: With this recipe, the ginger juice can warm the lungs and control cough, the juice of white radish can check the adverse effects of ascending qi, and control asthma. The honey can moisten the lungs and control cough.

Recipe 5: One-third fresh ginger and two-thirds taro.

Prescription: A paste of fresh ginger and taro is prepared after peeling and blending and then mixing in the same amount of wheat flour as ginger to prepare a thick paste. The paste is spread on a long piece of cloth or put into a cloth bag and then applied to the chest overnight for seven successive nights. By this method, asthma can be radically cured.

Explanation: This method can also produce specific effects to cure bronchial asthma.

Recipe 6: Fresh ginger 50 g and *baijiezi* (白 芥 子 , Seed of White Mustard) 15 g.

Prescription: The powder of *baijiezi* is mixed with ginger juice and alcohol to prepare a paste, and a gauze ball soaked with the paste is then used to rub the Dazhui (GV 14), Feishu (BL 13) and Danzhong (CV 17) acupoints for ten minutes at each acupoint to produce a local burning pain. As an alternative, a round folded piece of gauze, the size of a big coin, can be soaked with the paste and put on these three acupoints for one hour. When some pain is felt by the patient, the herbal paste gauze should be immediately taken away to avoid causing blisters.

Explanation: This method is more effective for treating patients with bronchial asthma in a shorter period of time.

Recipe 7: Ginger 50 g, walnut 50 g, bitter almond 50 g, and an adequate amount of honey.

Prescription: After peeling and soaking in water, the walnuts and almonds are pounded along with chopped ginger to make a paste; then mix with honey to prepare small pills for oral administration for ten nights.

Explanation: This recipe is used to treat cough with sputum

difficult to spit out due to heat in the lungs by nourishing and moistering the lungs.

Recipe 8: Fresh ginger juice 60 g, 5 pumpkins, and malt 1,500 g.

Prescription: After removing the seeds, the pumpkins are cut into pieces and well boiled in water until very soft. The clear pumpkin juice obtained by filtering and squeezing the boiled pumpkin with a piece of gauze is condensed by further boiling to one half its original quantity. The concentrated pumpkin juice is mixed with ginger juice and malt, and again boiled on a low flame to prepare a paste for oral administration of 150 g every night, or twice a day in severe cases.

Explanation: This recipe can control inflammation and pain, relieve toxicity, and treat chronic asthma.

5. Chronic Bronchitis

Recipe 1: Fresh ginger, green onion stalks, and *aiye* (艾 叶, Leaf of Mugwort) of an equal amount.

Prescription: The ingredients are boiled in water to prepare a decoction for oral administration.

Explanation: This recipe is used to treat chronic bronchitis caused by an attack of external wind and cold pathogens.

Recipe 2: Fresh ginger 60 g and mutton 250 g.

Prescription: The mutton is stewed with ginger as a dish for a meal.

Explanation: This method is used to treat chronic bronchitis of the deficient-cold type.

Recipe 3: Fresh ginger 15 g, almond 30 g, and honey 60 g.

Prescription: The ingredients are fried and then ground to prepare powder for oral administration, 10 g 2-3 times a day.

Explanation: This recipe is used to treat patients with chronic bronchitis and severe asthma.

Recipe 4: Fresh ginger 10 g and *aiye* (艾 叶, Leaf of Mugwort) 250 g.

Prescription: After steaming, the moxa (floccose *aiye*) and ginger are put into a cloth bag to be worn day and night until the disease is cured.

Explanation: This is a special method for treating chronic bronchitis.

Recipe 5: Fresh ginger 120 g, walnut 120 g, and brown sugar 120 g.

Prescription: The ingredients are pounded together to prepare a paste for oral administration of 9 g, 3 times a day.

Explanation: This preparation can produce good effects in treating chronic bronchitis.

Recipe 6: Several green onion stalks.

Prescription: After cutting into pieces, the green onion is put into a cloth bag and steamed for a hot compress placed over the throat and chest with the hot bag wrapped in a towel.

Explanation: This method is used to treat chronic bronchitis with sore throat, cough, and shortness of breath.

Recipe 7: Fresh ginger juice 5 ml, pear juice 50 ml, and *suye* (苏　叶, Leaf of Perilla) 6 g.

Prescription: The herb *suye* is boiled in water to prepare a decoction for oral administration twice a day after being mixed with ginger and pear juice.

Explanation: This recipe can warm the lungs and control cough and asthma.

Recipe 8: Fresh ginger juice 5 ml and *zhulishui* (竹 沥 水, Bamboo Juice) 30 ml.

Prescription: This is a dose for oral administration, 2-3 times a day.

Explanation: These ingredients can resolve sputum and control cough.

Recipe 9: Fresh ginger 10 g, sesame 30 g, and almond 12 g.

Prescription: The ingredients are boiled in water to prepare a decoction for oral administration, 2-3 times a day.

Explanation: This recipe can warm the lungs and control

cough and asthma due to an attack of wind and cold pathogens on the lungs.

Recipe 10: Fresh ginger 30 g and honey 500 g.

Prescription: Cut the ginger into slices, then put them into honey and steam for 20 minutes. After removing the ginger, 30-50 g of honey is orally administered, 1-2 times a day.

Explanation: This recipe is used to treat uncontrollable coughing and asthma caused by wind and dry pathogens.

Recipe 11: Fresh ginger 6 g and stem and leaf of eggplant 30 g.

Prescription: These ingredients are boiled in water to prepare a decoction for oral administration, 2-3 times a day.

Explanation: This is a recipe for treating uncontrollable cough and asthma.

Recipe 12: Twenty bulbs of garlic, lean pork 100 g, some salt, soybean sauce, and plant oil.

Prescription: The pork slices are fried in oil on a high flame with the peeled cloves of garlic for a while, and then mixed with the condiments as a dish for a meal.

Explanation: This preparation can control cough and resolve sputum to treat chronic bronchitis, but is not recommended for children.

Recipe 13: Ten bulbs of garlic, half a bowl of vinegar, and brown sugar 100 g.

Prescription: Garlic paste is mixed with sugar and then soaked in vinegar for 3 days. A vinegar extract of half a spoonful is drunk with warm boiled water, 3 times a day, after the garlic residue is removed.

Explanation: This preparation can produce a good therapeutic effect in treating chronic bronchitis, especially in aged patients.

6. Pulmonary Tuberculosis

Recipe 1: An adequate amount of garlic and sugar.

Prescription: The garlic slices are steamed with sugar for oral administration.

Explanation: Pulmonary tuberculosis is caused by an infection of tuberculous bacillus, usually in patients with a weak physique or a depletion of essence and qi in the body. Cough, hemoptysis, tidal fever, night sweating, weakness, chest pain, and pathological leanness are the main symptoms.

Recipe 2: Garlic with purple skin 15-20 cloves, *yimi* (薏 米 , Seed of Job's Tears) 30 g, and *baiji* (白 芨 , Bletilla) powder 4.5 g.

Prescription: The garlic is boiled in water and the garlic water is used to cook a rice soup of *yimi* mixed with half-cooked garlic and *baiji* powder for a meal once a day for 2 months.

Explanation: This preparation can nourish lung yin, clear up heat, and relieve toxicity to effectively treat pulmonary tuberculosis.

Recipe 3: Garlic with purple skin 15-20 cloves (about 20 g), rice 30 g, and *baiji* (白 芨 , Bletilla) powder 6.6 g.

Prescription: The peeled garlic is boiled in water for 1-1.5 minutes and the garlic water is used to cook a rice soup for 2 meals in one day, after mixing with boiled garlic and *baiji* powder.

Explanation: This recipe is used to treat pulmonary tuberculosis and its therapeutic effect may be further enhanced if *huangjing* (黄 精 , Sealwort) 45 g is added when cooking the rice soup.

Recipe 4: Garlic 15 g and one egg.

Prescription: The egg is stirred in boiled water and the warm egg soup is mixed with garlic paste for oral administration, twice a day.

Explanation: Sugar or salt may be added to the soup without disturbing its therapeutic effect.

Recipe 5: An adequate amount of garlic.

Prescription: The garlic is steamed in a jar. The patient is asked to inhale the hot steam, 3 times a day.

Recipe 6: Two bulbs of garlic, eel 150 g, and an adequate amount of green onion, ginger, plant oil, and salt.

Prescription: After removing viscera, washing and cutting into pieces, the eel is fried in oil until golden yellow and then boiled with garlic and condiments in water until the eel is well done.

Explanation: This preparation can inhibit the growth of tuberculous bacillus, heal consumption, and expel wind and damp pathogens.

Recipe 7: An adequate amount of garlic and vinegar.

Prescription: After soaking in vinegar for 7 days, 3 bulbs of garlic are taken twice a day over a long period of time.

Explanation: This recipe can promote blood circulation and produce a bactericidal effect. It can also be used to treat mild bronchitis and pulmonary tuberculosis.

Recipe 8: Fresh garlic, 4 cloves.

Prescription: The garlic may be taken after chewing well, 3-4 times a day or with meals.

Explanation: The garlic can relieve toxicity, control inflammation, and produce bacteriostatic and bactericidal effects to control infection.

Recipe 9: Fresh garlic juice 5 ml, fresh pear juice 50 ml, and fresh lotus root juice 30 ml.

Prescription: Mix the juice in above doses and then take once a day.

Explanation: The garlic juice may produce a strong effect to relieve toxicity and certain therapeutic effects in treating pulmonary tuberculosis. The pear and lotus root juice as a supplemental component of the recipe can increase body fluids and moisten the lungs.

Recipe 10: One bulb of garlic and 2 loach fish.

Prescription: Boil the ingredients in water and then eat the loaches and drink the soup once a day.

Explanation: The garlic can inhibit the growth of bacteria and the loach can supply nutrients. Therefore, this preparation can expel pathogens, improve nutrition, and reinforce the body's resistance.

7. Lung Abscess

Recipe 1: Garlic with purple skin 50 g and vinegar 100 g.

Prescription: The garlic paste is boiled in vinegar for about 10 minutes and taken after meals, twice a day.

Explanation: This preparation can control inflammation, produce a bactericidal effect, and promote drainage of pus in treating lung abscess.

Recipe 2: An adequate amount of garlic and aged vinegar.

Prescription: The garlic cloves are soaked in aged vinegar for a year and a small wine cup of vinegar is taken with meals or twice a day, in the morning and evening.

Explanation: This garlic-soaked vinegar is used to treat lung abscess because it can relieve toxicity and obstruction of the drainage of pus, and control inflammation.

Recipe 3: Garlic 500 g, *bailian* (白 蔹 , Japanese Ampelopsis) 30 g and *baiji* (白 芨 , Bletilla) 30 g.

Prescription: The herbs are boiled in a kettle with 3,000 ml of water, first on a high flame, and then simmered. A rubber tube 2-3 feet long is connected to the opening of the kettle and the patient inhales the steam from other end of the tube for 1-2 hours a day, once a day or every 2 days. The garlic is taken.

Explanation: This is a supplemental treatment for chronic lung abscess to shorten the course of therapy.

8. Heart Diseases

Recipe 1: Seven pieces of ripe green onion.

Prescription: Juice the green onion and then take with some sesame oil.

Explanation: This method is used to treat critical patients

with heart pain.

Recipe 2: Large and ripe ginger 5 g.
Prescription: A decoction of chopped ginger is taken.
Explanation: This is a method for treating the onset of acute heart pain.

Recipe 3: Fresh ginger 6 g, mung beans 30 g, and 1 tomato.
Prescription: The tomato is taken with a decoction of ginger and mung beans, 2-3 times a day.
Explanation: This recipe can be used to treat palpitations of the heart induced by a variety of causes.

Recipe 4: Fresh ginger 10 g, skin of banana 50 g, and crystalline sugar 20 g.
Prescription: A decoction of these ingredients is drunk twice a day.
Explanation: This is a supplemental treatment for rheumatic heart disease.

Recipe 5: Fresh ginger 3 slices, *longgu* (龙 骨, Fossil Fragments) 30 g, and *baiziren* (柏 子 仁, Seed of Oriental Arborvitae) 15 g.
Prescription: A decoction of these ingredients is taken twice a day.
Explanation: This recipe can tranquilize the mind and relieve the uneasiness in treating rheumatic heart disease.

Recipe 6: Fresh ginger juice 3 ml, lotus leaf juice 30 ml, and cucumber juice 30 ml.
Prescription: Mix these juices and then take 2-3 times a day.
Explanation: This recipe is used to treat coronary atherosclerotic heart disease.

Reccipe 7: Fresh ginger 3 slices, *banlangen* (板 蓝 根, Woad) 30 g, and water chestnut 20 g.
Prescription: A decoction of these ingredients is taken 2-3 times a day.
Explanation: This recipe is used to treat myocarditis.

Recipe 8: Fresh ginger 10 g, coriander 30 g, and *yuxingcao* (鱼腥草, Fishwort) 30 g.

Prescription: A decoction of these herbs is taken 2-3 times a day.

Explanation: This recipe is used to treat pulmonary heart disease.

9. Chest Pain

Recipe 1: One bulb of garlic, fresh ginger 3 g, and *chenpi* (陈皮, Dried Tangerine Peel) 20 g.

Prescription: A decoction of these ingredients is orally administered, 2-3 times a day.

Explanation: This recipe is used to treat pain and distension in the chest due to the stagnation of qi.

Recipe 2: Fresh ginger 30 g, *baijuhua* (白菊花, White Chrysanthemum) 15 g, and *tianguazi* (甜瓜子, Sweet Melon Seed) 6 g.

Prescription: A decoction of these ingredients is orally administered 1-2 times a day.

Explanation: This recipe is used to treat pain and distension in the chest due to an accumulation of heat and phlegm.

Recipe 3: Fresh ginger 30 g, *dingxiang* (丁香, Clove) 10 g, and sugar 250 g.

Prescription: The sugar is boiled with a small amount of water in an aluminum pot over a low flame until it becomes a thin syrup; then the chopped ginger and clove powder are added and further boiled to form a thick syrup which will not adhere to the finger when touched. The hot syrup forms a soft disc when it is poured into a dish and cooled. Before it hardens, the syrup disc is cut into 50 cubes, and 3-4 cubes are taken after each meal.

Explanation: In this recipe, the fresh ginger can warm the spleen and stomach and expel cold and the clove can warm the spleen and stomach and restore yang for treating chest pain caused by a cold pathogen.

Recipe 4: Stem of garlic 10 g, *chenpi* (陈 皮 , Dried Tangerine Peel) 10 g and *cheqianzi* (车 前 子 , Plantain Seed) 30 g placed in a cloth bag.

Prescription: A decoction of these herbs is orally administered 1-2 times a day.

Explanation: This recipe is used to treat pleuritis with pain in the chest wall.

Recipe 5: Two garlic bulbs, fresh ginger 8 g, Chinese Yam 60 g, and taro 60 g.

Prescription: The herbs are pounded together to prepare a paste for external application over the lesion.

Explanation: This recipe is used to treat pain in the heart, chest distress, and dull or paroxysmal severe pain of the chest due to coagulation of cold pathogen in the heart or blood vessels, accumulation of heat and fire pathogen, stagnation of qi, and phlegm.

10. Hypertension

Recipe 1: An adequate amount of sugar, vinegar, and garlic.

Prescription: One or two bulbs of garlic with a mixture of sugar and vinegar is taken each morning before breakfast.

Explanation: This mixture can reduce high blood pressure.

Recipe 2: Celery 100 g, 5 layers of onion, 5 cloves of garlic, 5 water chestnuts, and 1 tomato.

Prescription: These five ingredients are boiled in four bowls of water on a low flame until one bowl of soup is produced for oral administration before going to bed.

Explanation: This recipe may produce a quick effect to control hypertension. The garlic also can reduce serum cholesterol and high blood pressure.

11. Hypotension

Recipe: Ginger.

Prescription: Clean fresh ginger with the skin peeled may be taken.

Explanation: The intake of fresh ginger may produce a good effect to treat hypotension. Chewing 1 g of fresh ginger may raise systolic blood pressure by 1.5 kPa and diastolic pressure by 1.9 kPa on average. Ginger tea or a soup of vegetables, bean curd, pork or chicken with plenty of chopped ginger may produce a good effect in treating hypotension.

12. Vertigo

Recipe 1: Green onion stalks 7-10 pieces, 15 red dates, and a small amount of sugar.

Prescription: The green onion and dates are boiled in water for 15 minutes and the sugar is added to the decoction after filtration for oral administration before going to bed for several days, depending on the development of the disease.

Explanation: This recipe is used to treat vertigo in patients with neurasthenia and insomnia.

Recipe 2: One lump of fresh ginger, *fulonggan* (伏龙肝, Calcined Yellow Earth) 30 g, and lotus leaf 30 g.

Prescription: A decoction of these ingredients is orally administered 1-2 times a day.

Explanation: This recipe can be used to treat vertigo due to various causes.

Recipe 3: Fresh ginger 6 g, *huangbo* (黄柏, Cork Tree) 10 g, and *digupi* (地骨皮, Matrimony Vine) 30 g.

Prescription: A decoction of these herbs is orally administered 1-2 times a day.

Explanation: This recipe is used to treat vertigo due to diseases of the inner ear.

13. Hyperlipemia

Recipe 1: Green onion 30 g and spinach 50 g.

Prescription: These two vegetables are fried to cook a dish

for 1-2 meals a day.

Explanation: This method can reduce serum cholesterol to prevent astherosclerosis.

Recipe 2: Fresh ginger 4 slices, *huoxiang* (霍 香 , Giant Hyssop) 6 g, and lotus leaf 15 g.

Prescription: The decoction of these herbs are orally administered 2-3 times a day.

Explanation: Acromatic herb can produce a dispersing function to reduce blood lipids.

Recipe 3: One bulb of garlic and 2 cucumbers.

Prescription: The cucumber slices are mixed with garlic paste for a vegetable salad eaten with 1-2 meals a day.

Explanation: The consistent intake of this salad over a long period of time may prevent the development of hyperlipemia.

14. Stomachache

Recipe 1: Ginger 5 slices, one pig tripe, and 10 grains of pepper.

Prescription: After washing clean with vinegar, the pig tripe is steamed with ginger slices and pepper and cooked until the tripe becomes very soft, then eaten for the morning and evening meals.

Explanation: This preparation is used to treat patients with chronic stomachache, weak physique, and poor appetite and weight loss.

Recipe 2: Fresh ginger 50 g, pig tripe 200 g, and cassia bark 5 g.

Prescription: After washing clean, the tripe is cut into slivers and steamed with ginger and cassia bark until it becomes soft for oral administration twice a day.

Explanation: This recipe is used to treat patients with dull pain in the upper abdomen, regurgitation of clear fluid, and loss of taste due to a deficiency of spleen and stomach yang, and cold pathogen in the spleen and stomach, because it can tone the spleen and stomach.

Recipe 3: Seven pieces of fresh garlic with leaves and an adequate amount of salt and vinegar.

Prescription: The fresh garlic is cut into bits and boiled with salt and vinegar as a hot soup for oral administration during an attack of stomachache.

Explanation: This preparation can promote the circulation of qi and stop the pain of stomachache.

Recipe 4: Dried ginger 10 g and 10 grains of pepper.

Prescription: After being sun-dried and pounded into a powder, the mixture of these two ingredients is taken twice a day.

Explanation: This powder can strengthen the stomach and expel cold pathogen to treat pain and cold in the stomach.

Recipe 5: One pig tripe and an adequate amount of ripe ginger.

Prescription: The ginger sliced to the thickness of a coin is combined with the tripe and thoroughly steamed until it is very soft. The tripe with the broth is divided into 2 portions and taken twice a day.

Explanation: Ginger with its warm nature can expel cold pathogen, relieve exterior syndrome, and control vomiting to treat cold and pain in the stomach. It can also stimulate the stomach nerves to promote peristalsis of the stomach and stimulate the small intestines to improve the absorption of chyliferous vessels. Pig tripe also can strengthen the stomach.

Recipe 6: An adequate amount of ripe ginger.

Prescription: After drying and baking over a low fire, the ginger is cut into small bits and taken with breakfast in the morning.

Explanation: The ginger is used to treat cold and pain in the stomach. While ginger is being used for treatment, bananas, papaya, rice noodles, and fresh or pickled Chinese cabbage must be avoided.

Recipe 7: Ripe ginger 500 g and crystal sugar 100 g.

Prescription: The unwashed ginger is put into the ash of burned charcoal or firewood. On the second morning the burned skin is removed and the intact central portion of the ginger is cut into thin slices and stored in a sealed jar with the powder of crystal sugar for 1 week, until the sugar is well-mixed with and absorbed by the ginger. The ginger is chewed well and then swallowed, 2-4 times a day.

Explanation: This preparation can be used to treat stomachache due to gastric and duodenal ulcers or other causes. The stomachache may be cured by this treatment in one month in mild cases, and in half a year in severe cases.

Recipe 8: Green onion stalks 10 g, fresh ginger 6 g, pepper 3 g, and *bingpian* (冰 片 , Borneol) 2 g.

Prescription: A powder made of these ingredients is mixed with sesame oil and wheat flour to prepare a paste for external application to the umbilical region.

Explanation: This method is used to treat stomachache of the deficient-cold type due to endogenous cold in the spleen and stomach.

Recipe 9: Green onion stalks 20 g, *aiye* (艾 叶 , Leaf of Mugwort) 20 g, cactus 20 g, and salt 20 g.

Prescription: A hot paste made of these ingredients is applied over the epigastric area and lower abdomen.

Explanation: This method is used to treat stomachache caused by stagnation of food in the stomach.

Recipe 10: Fresh ginger 3,500 g, brown sugar 2,500 g and *sharen* (砂 仁 , Grains of Paradise) 500 g.

Prescription: A paste made from these ingredients is stored in a jar and buried in the earth for 10 days. It is then orally administered with water in a dosage of 50 g.

Explanation: This aromatic preparation can treat stomachache of various causes by strengthening the stomach.

Recipe 11: Fresh ginger 25 g, Chinese chives 250 g, and milk

250 g.

Prescription: The ginger is washed clean and pounded, and the Chinese chives are cut and squeezed to produce juice. The juice of the ginger and Chinese chives are mixed and boiled with milk to prepare a hot drink.

Explanation: This preparation is used to treat stomachache due to stagnation of cold pathogen in the stomach with a sudden onset of pain, exacerbated by cold, and relieved by hot in patients preferring hot food and drink.

Recipe 12: Dried ginger 9 g and *zhigancao* (炙 甘 草, Honey-fried Licorice) 15 g.

Prescription: A decoction of these two herbs is for oral administration.

Explanation: This recipe is used to treat epigastric pain caused by cold in the stomach.

15. Peptic Stomach Ulcer

Recipe 1: Fresh ginger 250 g and one pig tripe.

Prescription: The ginger is put into well-washed tripe with its openings ligated and then boiled in an earthenware pot on a low fire. After removing the ginger, the tripe is cut into slivers with soybean sauce for oral administration and the soup is drunk. One tripe is taken over three days, and the treatment is continued for one month.

Explanation: Besides peptic stomach ulcers, this method can also be used to treat stomachache due to an attack of cold pathogen.

Recipe 2: One chicken (over 500 g) and large fresh ginger 250 g.

Prescription: After removing the viscera and washed clean, the chicken is steamed for about two and a half hours with about two small bowls of ginger juice filled in the body cavity. The chicken soup with ginger juice is taken.

Explanation: The soup is more useful for treating peptic

ulcer, although the meat may be taken at the same time. The disease may be cured and health improved after treatment with about five chickens.

16. Hyperhydrochloria

Recipe: Garlic 50 g and lean pork meat 150-200 g.

Prescription: The garlic and pork are steamed a little over half an hour for oral administration.

Explanation: This method is used to treat hyperhydrochloria with regurgitation of sour fluid.

17. Chronic Gastritis

Recipe 1: Rice 100 g and an adequate amount of ginger juice.

Prescription: After soaking in water, the rice is wrapped in 5-6 sheets of linen paper and burned into ash. After grinding, the fine powder of burned rice is taken with ginger juice, twice a day. For mild cases, one preparation of rice ash is enough; severe cases need three preparations. In the first week of treatment, the patients should take only liquid food. Uncooked, cold or greasy food is prohibited.

Explanation: This is an effective method for treating chronic gastritis, especially useful for mild cases in a shorten course of treatment.

Recipe 2: Fresh ginger 20 g and orange peel 20 g.

Prescription: A decoction of these ingredients is taken 2-3 times a day.

Explanation: This recipe is useful for treating chronic gastritis with stomachache and vomiting of mucus and clear fluid because of its ability to strengthen the stomach and relieve toxicity.

18. Vomiting

Recipe 1: A soupspoon of fresh ginger juice and half a cup of sugar cane juice.

Prescription: The mixed juice obtained by pounding and squeezing the ginger and cane is prepared for oral administration.

Explanation: This juice can clear heat, relieve toxicity and adjust the stomach to treat vomiting with or without vomitus due to stomach cancer at the early stage. It can also relieve pregnancy reactions and chronic stomach diseases.

Recipe 2: Fresh ginger 50 g and one piece of fruit candy.

Prescription: Before travel, the clean ginger is chewed and then swallowed, and a piece of fruit candy is sucked.

Explanation: This method can strengthen the stomach and stop vomiting to prevent dizziness, vertigo, nausea, and vomiting caused by all forms of motion sickness.

Recipe 3: Fresh ginger, white pepper, and *zisu* (紫 苏 , Leaf of Perilla) 5 g of each.

Prescription: A decoction of these herbs is taken.

Explanation: This recipe can strengthen the stomach to treat vomiting and abdominal pain due to indigestion and stagnation of greasy food.

Recipe 4: An adequate amount of garlic and mutton.

Prescription: Some boiled mutton is taken with garlic at will.

Explanation: These ingredients can be used to treat vomiting.

Recipe 5: Fresh ginger 60 g and an adequate amount of brown sugar and vinegar.

Prescription: The clean ginger slices are soaked in vinegar for one day. Three slices of ginger are put in boiled water with some brown sugar to make a cup of tea for drinking.

Explanation: This method is used to treat nausea, vomiting, poor appetite, and stomachache due to an attack of cold pathogen.

Recipe 6: Fresh ginger 100 g and *sharen* (砂 仁 , Grains of Paradise) 5 g.

Prescription: After washing, cutting, and pounding, the ginger paste is wrapped in a piece of gauze and the ginger juice is squeezed out. The ginger juice and *sharen* are put in half a bowl of water and steamed for half an hour. After removing the dregs, the decoction is taken.

Explanation: This recipe is used to treat vomiting due to cold in the stomach, abdominal pain, and pregnancy vomiting.

Recipe 7: Fresh ginger 20 g and fresh *zisuye* (紫 苏 叶 , Leaf of Perilla) 30 g.

Prescription: The juice obtained by pounding these two herbs is taken with warm water.

Explanation: This method is used to treat vomiting after an attack of coolness.

Recipe 8: Fresh ginger 50 g and honey 25 g.

Prescription: The ginger juice and honey are well-mixed and slightly steamed or boiled for oral administration with warm water.

Explanation: This method is used to treat nausea and vomiting.

Recipe 9: Fresh ginger 50 g and *shichangpu* (石 菖 蒲 , Rock Sweetflag) 15 g.

Prescription: After washing and pounding, the juice of these two herbs is obtained for oral administration with warm water.

Explanation: This recipe is used to treat vomiting due to a disturbance in the stomach's transporting function.

Recipe 10: Fresh ginger 10 g, hawthorn 10 g, and fresh soybean sauce 15 ml.

Prescription: A decoction of these ingredients is taken 1-2 times a day.

Explanation: The ginger can warm the spleen and stomach to stop vomiting, and the hawthorn can improve digestion and control vomiting.

Recipe 11: Fresh ginger three slices, one potato, and one orange.

Prescription: After peeling the skin, the orange is pounded with the potato and ginger to prepare a paste for oral administration, one spoonful of paste 2-3 times a day.

Explanation: This method is used to treat vomiting due to the blockage of the transportation of qi.

Recipe 12: Fresh ginger 10 g, a segment of bamboo, and *suye* (苏 叶, Leaf of Persilla) 6 g.

Prescription: A decoction of these herbs is orally administered, 1-2 times a day.

Explanation: This recipe can suppress the adverse ascent of qi to treat vomiting due to an adverse ascent of stomach qi.

Recipe 13: Fresh ginger 50 g and fresh lotus root 250 g.

Prescription: The clean ginger and lotus root are pounded and squeezed to prepare juice in a quantity for oral administration, 1-2 times a day for 3 days.

Explanation: This method is used to stop vomiting and hematemesis.

Recipe 14: Fresh ginger 20 g.

Prescription: The ginger is pounded to prepare juice for oral administration with warm water.

Explanation: The ginger can expel cold pathogen to treat vomiting caused by the accumulation of cold pathogen in the stomach.

19. Hematemesis

Recipe: Ginger charcoal 9 g, *baiji* (白 芨 , Bletilla) 30 g, and *fulonggan* (伏 龙 肝, Caleined Yellow Earth) 60 g.

Prescription: The powder of ginger charcoal and *baiji* is orally administered with a decoction of *fulonggan*, 2-3 times a day.

Explanation: Hematemesis is the vomiting of blood due to bleeding in the upper digestive tract. Sometimes, it is dark purple in color and mixed with undigested food.

20. Hiccups

Recipe 1: Fresh ginger 6 g and orange peel 3 g.

Prescription: A decoction of these ingredients is taken 1-2

times a day.

Explanation: This is a useful method for treating nausea, hiccups, and cold limbs.

Recipe 2: Fresh ginger 3 g.

Prescription: An attack of hiccups can be quickly controlled by drinking hot tea made with ginger bits.

Explanation: This method is used to treat continuous hiccups due to an attack of cold in the stomach or a disorder of liver qi.

Recipe 3: Equal amounts of fresh ginger, calyx of persimmon, and granulated sugar.

Prescription: A hot concentrated decoction of these ingredients is orally administered.

Explanation: This is a useful method for controlling hiccups due to the adverse ascent of qi.

Recipe 4: Fresh ginger juice 5 ml and juice of white radish 30 ml.

Prescription: The mixed juice of these ingredients is prepared for one drink, 1-2 times a day.

Explanation: Both ginger juice and the juice of white radish can suppress hiccups and the adverse ascent of qi, and control vomiting.

21. Jaundice

Recipe: Fresh ginger 9 g, *digupi* (地 骨 皮 , Chinese Wolf-Berry Root Bark) 9 g, and *aiye* (艾 叶 , Leaf of Mugwort) 3 g.

Prescription: A 20 ml concentrated decoction of these herbs, with an adequate amount of vinegar, is administered orally, 2-3 times a day.

Explanation: Jaundice is usually caused by viral hepatitis or other diseases such as cirrhosis of the liver, leptospirosis, and diseases of the biliary tract. The eyes, skin, and urine become yellow in color.

22. Hepatitis

Recipe: Garlic 50 g.

Prescription: Garlic paste is taken with mung bean soup and a small amount of sugar, twice a day.

Explanation: Together with other medicinal therapy and improved nutrition, this decoction can be used to treat chronic hepatitis.

23. Cirrhosis of Liver

Recipe: Garlic onion (with roots and leaves) 120 g and sodium sulfate 60 g.

Prescription: After heating in a pot over a low flame, a hot paste of these ingredients is wrapped in a piece of gauze and applied over the umbilicus, together with a hot water bag to maintain the warmth of the paste, for 3 hours.

Explanation: This method is used to treat patients with cirrhosis of the liver, ascites, and retention of urine and stool.

24. Kidney Stone

Recipe 1: Fresh green onion 250 g and one pig's foot.

Prescription: The pig's foot is boiled with green onion, including roots, until very soft and the soup is taken to promote urination. The kidney stone may be passed after drinking this soup for 3 days and the disease may be cured after continuous treatment with this method.

Explanation: This is one metbod for treating kidney stone. The pig's foot may or may not be eaten with the soup.

Recipe 2: Fine green onion 250 g, lean pork meat 250 g, an adequate amount of starch, and a small amount of salt.

Prescription: The minced pork meat is mixed with starch and salt, and placed on the fine green onion, spread over the bottom of a pot for boiling with an adequate amount of water until the meat is well done as a dish for a meal with rice, once a day. The soup and onion should be taken at the same time.

Explanation: The kidney stone may be dissolved and discharged after using this treatment for one to two weeks.

25. Abdominal Mass

Recipe 1: An adequate amount of garlic and vinegar.

Prescription: The vinegar and the soaked garlic are taken.

Explanation: This method is used to treat abdominal masses, and masses containing blood in women.

Recipe 2: An adequate amount of single-clove garlic.

Prescription: The intake of boiled single-clove garlic alone or with other food over a long period of time may generate the resolution of masses in the body.

Explanation: This method is used to treat masses over a long period of time.

Recipe 3: A few inches of green onion stalks and honey 30 g.

Prescription: A paste made of these two ingredients is applied over the mass and, after covering with a piece of cloth, the lesion is stroked with a hot iron.

Explanation: This method is used to treat food stagnation and masses containing blood.

26. Abdominal Distention

Recipe 1: Several bulbs of garlic and granulated sugar 250 g.

Prescription: The garlic is well boiled with sugar until it is very soft for oral administration.

Explanation: This method is used to treat ascites. Salt is prohibited for three years to patients using this method.

Recipe 2: An adequate amount of single-clove garlic.

Prescription: The hot stewed garlic with skin peeled is wrapped with silk floss and put into the anus. When the first application cools, it is replaced with new hot garlic.

Explanation: This method is used to treat abdominal distention.

Recipe 3: Five bulbs of garlic with skin peeled, 4 large snails, and *cheqianzi* (车 前 子 , Plantain Seed) powder 9 g.

Prescription: A paste made by grinding these ingredients together is applied into the umbilicus and covered by a handkerchief for a while. Urine soon may be discharged.

Explanation: This method is used to treat edema and abdominal distention.

27. Abdominal Pain

Recipe 1: Baked ginger 1 g and *wulingzhi* (五 灵 脂 , Bat Dung) 4 g.

Prescription: A powder of these ingredients is taken with hot rice wine.

Explanation: This is used for abdominal pain actually located below the epigastric region and above the pubic symphysis.

Recipe 2: Garlic paste 6 g, fresh ginger 6 g, and sugar 12 g.

Prescription: A powder of these ingredients is taken with water.

Explanation: This recipe is used to treat abdominal pain due to an attack of cold pathogen.

Recipe 3: Dried ginger 3 g, *rougui* (肉 桂 , Cassia Bark) 1.5 g, and *fuzi* (附 子 , Monkshood) 15 g.

Prescription: A decoction of these ingredients is orally administered.

Explanation: This recipe is used to treat abdominal pain due to an attack of cold pathogen.

Recipe 4: Fresh ginger 100 g and vinegar 250 ml.

Prescription: The clean ginger slivers are soaked in vinegar and stored in a tight container. The ginger vinegar in an amount of 10 ml is taken before a meal once a day.

Explanation: This preparation may be stored at home for emergency usage in treating abdominal pain due to an attack of cold pathogen.

Recipe 5: Fresh ginger 100 g, garlic 100 g, and vinegar 50

ml.

Prescription: The clean slices of fresh ginger and garlic cloves are soaked in vinegar and stored in a sealed container for one month before consuming.

Explanation: This method is used to treat abdominal pain due to an attack of cold pathogen or from eating too much fruits.

Recipe 6: Garlic 1,500 g.

Prescription: The garlic is soaked in a mixture of vinegar and liquor for 10 days for oral administration, 3-5 bulbs of garlic a day for one week.

Recipe 7: An adequate amount of fresh ginger and green onion.

Prescription: The paste of ginger and green onion is taken with some hot wine. The patient then may have a nap to induce sweating and the abdominal pain may be quickly relieved. If the abdominal pain is very severe, the paste of onion is applied over the umbilicus with moxibustion and the pain may be relieved.

Explanation: This method is used to treat abdominal pain caused by an attack of cold pathogen during sexual intercourse.

Recipe 8: Ten bulbs of garlic and an adequate amount of vinegar and liquor.

Prescription: The garlic is soaked in a mixture of vinegar and liquor for 2-3 years. When ready for use, 1-2 bulbs of soaked garlic is taken. Boiled garlic may be taken as a substitute.

Explanation: This method can promote the circulation of qi in treating abdominal pain due to emotional disturbance and stagnation of qi.

28. Dysentery

Recipe 1: Fresh ginger 9 g and 2 eggs.

Prescription: A steamed egg with pounded ginger is taken before meals, twice a day.

Explanation: The fresh ginger with its pungent odor and

warm nature can relieve exterior syndrome and expel pathogens, and the egg with its sweet taste and moist properties can relieve toxicity and reinforce the body's resistance. This is an appropriate method for treating dysentery in the early stages with fever and chills.

Recipe 2: Two bulbs of single-clove garlic and one egg.

Prescription: The egg is fried in a pan with garlic until the garlic becomes soft for oral administration before meals over a long period of time until the dysentery is cured.

Explanation: The garlic can relieve toxicity in treating dysentery, and the egg can adjust the functions of the spleen and stomach. Therefore, this is a good dietary therapy for dysentery, combining the therapeutic effects of both ginger and egg.

Recipe 3: An adequate amount of dried ginger.

Prescription: The dried ginger is baked until it starts turning blacks, maintaining its pharmacological properties, and 5 g of baked ginger powder is then taken with rice gruel to produce a good therapeutic result.

Explanation: This method is used to treat acute dysentery with blood in the stools.

Recipe 4: Ginger juice 15 g, turnip juice 60 g, honey 30 g, and a cup of concentrated tea.

Prescription: A mixture of these juices is boiled or steamed for one oral administration.

Explanation: The ginger can reinforce stomach and intestine functions, relieve toxicity, and produce a bactericidal effect in treating dysentery when used with other ingredients. This method is especially useful in treating dysentery patients with tenesmus.

Recipe 5: Two garlic bulbs.

Prescription: The chopped garlic is boiled with an adequate amount of rice to prepare a thin paste for oral administration. The garlic may be soaked in vinegar and sugar to prepare the sweet and sour garlic for administration.

Explanation: The garlic can promote digestion and produce a strong bactericidal effect in treating bacterial infection.

Recipe 6: One garlic bulb and sugar 20 g.

Prescription: The chopped garlic is mixed with sugar for oral administration before meals every morning and evening for 7-10 days.

Explanation: This method is used to treat bacillary dysentery and enteritis with diarrhea because the garlic can relieve toxicity and kill bacteria. For bacillary dysentery an enema with garlic fluid may produce a good therapeutic effect.

Recipe 7: One bulb of garlic, three-colored amaranth 100 g, and a small amount of sesame oil.

Prescription: After washing and cutting, the amaranth is fried in sesame oil on a high flame and then mixed with garlic paste for oral administration.

Explanation: This method is used to treat bacillary dysentery, but the amaranth should not be fried for a long time, otherwise the effective component may be destroyed and the therapeutic effect may be reduced.

Recipe 8: Fresh ginger 6 g, brown sugar 30 g, and fine tea leaves 15 g.

Prescription: These ingredients are put in a cup to make half a cup of tea with boiled water. After the tea has been drunk, another half cup of tea may be taken as one treatment. In severe cases, this tea may be drunk twice a day.

Explanation: The tea can produce a bactericidal and astringent effect for treating bacillary dysentery with blood and pus in stools and acute enteritis with diarrhea.

Recipe 9: Two bulbs of garlic and a small amount of white and brown sugar.

Prescription: The garlic paste is soaked in an adequate amount of boiled water for 4 hours and the filtrate is mixed with sugar for oral administration.

Explanation: The garlic can produce a bactericidal and antiscolic effect in treating dysentery with good therapeutic results. Fresh garlic in the amount of 6 g can be taken once a day for 10 days to treat amebic dysentery.

Recipe 10: Fresh ginger 5 slices, one quail, and red beans 30 g.

Prescription: Cubes of quail are boiled with red beans and ginger to prepare a soup for oral administration, twice a day.

Explanation: Besides its therapeutic effect in treating dysentery with blood and pus in stools, this soup is also a nourishing food to tone the internal organs.

Recipe 11: One bulb of single-clove garlic and green tea 60 g.

Prescription: The green tea and garlic paste are put in a teapot to make tea with boiled water for constant drinking.

Explanation: This is a useful method of treating chronic bacillary dysentery, but the tea should be drunk constantly for a long time.

Recipe 12: A garlic suspension 10 percent or extract 70-100 ml.

Prescription: The garlic suspension or extract is used for a retention enema once a day for 6 days as a therapeutic course. At the same time, a bulb of fresh garlic with purple skin is divided into 3 portions for 3 oral administration.

Explanation: This method can produce a bacteriostatic and pesticidal effect and relieve toxicity in treating amebic dysentery.

Recipe 13: Two bulbs of garlic and fried hawthorn 30 g.

Prescription: A decoction is made by these two ingredients and taken 2-3 times a day.

Explanation: This method is used to treat indigestion and uncontrollable diarrhea.

Recipe 14: Fresh ginger 6 g, *chenpi* (陈 皮, Dried Tangerine Peel) 10 g, and apple peel 20 g.

Prescription: A decoction is made by these ingredients and

taken 2-3 times a day.

Explanation: This method is used to treat dysentery due to stagnation of turbid dampness in the spleen and stomach.

Recipe 15: An adequate amount of garlic with purple skin.

Prescription: One bulb of garlic with purple skin is divided into 3 portions for oral administration, 3 times a day. A retention enema using a 10 percent garlic suspension of 70-100 ml is administered every night. After the disease is cured, the intake of one half to one bulb of fresh garlic with purple skin, once a day, should be continued for 1-2 months to prevent a relapse of dysentery.

Explanation: This method is used to treat amebic dysentery, an infectious disease of the digestive tract caused by ameba infection. Patients may have abdominal pain, low fever and diarrhea, and may pass gellike stools with a foul odor many times a day.

29. Febrile Infectious Diseases

Recipe 1: Three pieces of tender leaf of green onion 1.6 cm, and a pinch of sugar.

Prescription: The green onion and sugar are mixed and pounded to prepare a paste for application to the palms, soles, and philtrum of the sick baby. The baby is then totally and tightly wrapped in a blanket, except for the nose and mouth, for one hour.

Explanation: The treatment should continue even if the baby cries and struggles. A layer of sticky sweat with a foul odor may appear all over the baby's body after the blanket is removed. The baby may have a bath after the fever is under control.

Recipe 2: Fresh ginger 50 g, 10 green onion stalks, and 2 bowls of wine.

Prescription: The ginger and green onion are boiled in wine until one bowl of hot decoction is obtained for oral administration to induce sweating while the patient is covered with a heavy blanket. Symptoms may be quickly relieved after moderate sweating.

Explanation: The sweating should not be profused, and greasy food should be avoided for 5-7 days.

30. Cholera

Recipe 1: An adequate amount of ginger slices and salt.

Prescription: A preparation of salt between two slices of ginger is used to rub the chest with some water. This treatment may be continued for 15 minutes. And then the part above the sacrum is rubbed for another 15 minutes.

Explanation: This method can be used to treat cholera with uncontrollable vomiting and diarrhea.

Recipe 2: Garlic 20-30 cloves.

Prescription: A garlic paste is prepared and applied over both soles.

Explanation: This method is used to treat cholera with critical symptoms such as abdominal colic and spasms of the calf muscles.

Recipe 3: Small garlic 250 g.

Prescription: The garlic is boiled in 2 liters of water until 1 litre of decoction is obtained for constant drinking.

Explanation: This method is used to treat choleroid diseases with abdominal distention, nausea, and constipation.

Recipe 4: Fresh ginger 90 g.

Prescription: The pounded ginger is boiled in 500 ml of wine for one oral administration.

Explanation: This method is used to treat uncontrollable diarrhea, abdominal pain, and muscle spasms.

Recipe 5: Ginger 30 g and *douchi* (豆 豉, Medicated Soybean) 60 g.

Prescription: These herbs are pounded to prepare a powder which is then divided into 2 portions. After heating in a pot, it is used to rub the umbilical region.

Explanation: This method is used to treat abdominal colic pain in choleroid diseases.

Recipe 6: Ripe ginger 50 g and *shichangpu* (石 菖 蒲 , Rock Sweetflag) 15 g.

Prescription: After washing, the herbs are pounded to prepare a juice for oral administration with water, twice a day.

Explanation: This preparation can adjust the stomach and control vomiting and diarrhea in choleroid diseases.

31. Diarrhea

Recipe 1: An adequate amount of garlic and sugar.
Prescription: Bake the garlic and eat it with sugar.
Explanation: This method is used to treat chronic diarrhea.

Recipe 2: Two bulbs of garlic.

Prescription: The garlic bulbs are roasted until the skins turns black. They are then boiled with an adequate amount of water to prepare a fluid for oral administration.

Explanation: The garlic can kill bacteria and improve digestive functions in treating diarrhea with foul stools.

Recipe 3: An equal amount of garlic and *dandouchi* (淡 豆 豉 , Medicated Soybean).

Prescription: These herbs are mixed and ground to prepare small pills the size of the seeds of the Chinese parasol tree for oral administration. Thirty pills each time.

Explanation: This preparation is used to treat abdominal pain and chronic diarrhea with blood in stool. Administration should continue for one month, and the disease may be cured.

Recipe 4: Garlic 15-25 g and purslane 50-100 g.

Prescription: The purslane is boiled in water to prepare a bowl of hot decoction that is then poured into the garlic paste and well-mixed. The filtrated potion is divided into 2 portions for oral administration with sugar, twice a day.

Explanation: The garlic can produce a bactericidal and

anti-inflammatory effect to treat diarrhea due to gastroenteritis. The scorched garlic with its therapeutic effect intact may be taken 2.5-5.0 g, 2-3 times a day to produce a good therapeutic result.

Recipe 5: Fresh ginger 15 g, 3 eggs, vinegar 15 ml, and some green onion and salt.
Prescription: The ginger bits, green onion, and salt are mixed with the beatened eggs to prepare a fried egg cake as a dessert for oral administration after roasting with vinegar. This dessert may be taken repeatedly until symptoms are improved.
Explanation: This method can be used to treat chronic diarrhea due to cold accumulated in the spleen and stomach.

Recipe 6: An adequate amount of garlic and vinegar.
Prescription: The garlic cloves are soaked in vinegar and preserved for use. During an attack of vomiting and diarrhea, 6 cloves of soaked garlic are taken, 3 times a day.
Explanation: This method can also be used to treat enteritis. The soaked garlic may be continually taken to prevent infectious diseases of the digestive tract.

Recipe 7: Several cloves of garlic.
Prescription: A mixture of garlic paste and vinegar in a winecup may be slowly sipped.
Explanation: This is a simple method to effectively treat gastroenteritis.

Recipe 8: An adequate amount of green onion.
Prescription: A paste of green onion is mixed with yellow lead to prepare pills in the size of a soybean for application in the umbilicus, which is then covered with a piece of herbal adhesive plaster.
Explanation: This is a useful method for treating stubborn chronic diarrhea.

Recipe 9: Two lumps of fresh ginger and a handful of *aiye* (艾 叶 , Leaf of Mugwort).
Prescription: These herbs is decocted with one bowl of water

and then administered orally, twice a day.

Explanation: The fresh ginger can expel cold pathogen and warm the spleen and stomach, and the mugwort can warm the meridians and release stagnation in the meridians for treating diarrhea of the cold-deficient type.

Recipe 10: An adequate amount of ginger juice and liquor and a sticky rice ball (pyramid shaped).

Prescription: The sticky rice ball is cut into slices and sundried. After steaming, 100 g of the sticky rice slices are taken with some ginger juice and liquor, twice a day.

Explanation: This method can warm and nourish the spleen and stomach and expel cold pathogen for treating patients with pale lips, insensitive taste buds, and diarrhea with clear watery stools.

Recipe 11: Green onion 100 g and some salt.

Prescription: The green onion and salt are fried and wrapped in a cloth bag for application as a hot compress to the abdomen, back, and waist.

Explanation: This method can expel cold pathogen and warm the spleen and stomach for treating abdominal pain and diarrhea caused by cold pathogen.

Recipe 12: Fresh ginger 10 g.

Prescription: The fresh ginger is baked over a low flame and then ground to prepare a powder for oral administration of 1 g, twice a day. The baked ginger powder may be administered with ginger juice for babies.

Explanation: This preparation can expel cold in treating diarrhea and indigestion caused by cold pathogen.

Recipe 13: Green onion stalks 20 g, leaves of the heaven tree (Folium Ailanthus altissima) 20 g, *aiye* (艾 叶, Leaf of Mugwort) 20 g, and salt 20 g.

Prescription: A hot decoction of these herbs is made and used to wash the feet, twice a day.

Explanation: This method can clear heat, eliminate dampness, stop diarrhea, and control pain for treating acute diarrhea caused by heat and damp pathogens.

Recipe 14: Fresh ginger 6 g, garlic 12 g, *fulonggan* (伏 龙 肝, Calcined Yellow Earth) 30 g, and 12 pieces of dates.

Prescription: A paste of these herbs is made and applied over the abdomen or umbilical region, followed by moxibustion over the paste.

Explanation: This method can warm the spleen and stomach for treating severe diarrhea caused by cold pathogen.

Recipe 15: Fresh ginger 3 g, fine tea leaves 6 g, brown sugar 20 g, and peel of pomelo.

Prescription: These herbs are boiled to prepare a paste for oral administration, twice a day.

Explanation: This recipe can warm the spleen and stomach and eliminate dampness for treating chronic diarrhea caused by cold and damp pathogens.

Recipe 16: Three bulbs of single-clove garlic, one sweet potato, and brown sugar 30 g.

Prescription: The garlic and brown sugar are put into the sweet potato and then roasted for oral administration.

Explanation: This preparation can nourish spleen qi for treating chronic diarrhea due to spleen deficiency.

Recipe 17: Green onion 60 g, *wubeizi* (五 倍 子, Chinese Galnut) 30 g and *aiye* (艾 叶, Leaf of Mugwort) 20 g.

Prescription: A powder of these herbs is mixed with sesame oil or vaseline to prepare a paste for external application over the abdomen.

Explanation: This preparation can expel cold pathogen for treating chronic diarrhea caused by cold and damp pathogens.

Recipe 18: An adequate amount of garlic and pepper.

Prescription: A powder of these two ingredients is used to make small cakes for application over the umbilicus or soles of the feet.

Explanation: This method is used to treat abdominal pain

and diarrhea with watery stools due to an attack of cold pathogen.

Recipe 19: Fresh ginger 3 g, pepper 14 grains, and *dandouchi* (淡豆豉, Medicated Soybean) 6 g.

Prescription: A hot decoction of these herbs is orally administered.

Explanation: This recipe is used to treat abdominal pain, cold limbs, and diarrhea caused by cold pathogen.

Recipe 20: Fresh ginger 9 g and dry rice flour cake 30 g.

Prescription: The ginger is put into the rice flour cake and soaked in boiled water until the cake becomes soft for oral administration.

Explanation: The fresh ginger can warm the body and expel cold accumulation for treating abdominal pain and diarrhea due to an attack of cold pathogen.

Recipe 21: Three bulbs of garlic with skin peeled and then pounded to prepare a paste, and 2 eggs.

Prescription: The eggs are fried with garlic paste for oral administration, twice a day.

Explanation: This method is used in treating diarrhea in weak patients.

Recipe 22: Tea leaves 100 g and dried ginger 50 g.

Prescription: A mixed powder of these two ingredients is taken. Five g, 2-3 times a day.

Explanation: This method is used in treating diarrhea with tenesmus and foul stools due to an attack of heat and damp pathogens.

32. Indigestion

Recipe 1: Fresh ginger 6 g and areca nut 9 g.

Prescription: A decoction of these herbs is orally administered, twice a day.

Explanation: This recipe can improve appetite, strengthen the spleen, and expel parasites.

Recipe 2: An adequate amount of fresh ginger and *zisu* (紫 苏 , Leave of Perilla).

Prescription: After soaking the hand in hot decoction of these herbs for a while, the hot hand is then used to rub the precordial and abdominal region to improve digestion. The hot dregs of the decoction is wrapped in a cloth bag for a hot compress to the chest and abdomen. The decoction is kept hot over a flame and the hot compress bag is repeatedly immersed in it for use.

Explanation: This method is used to treat indigestion due to cold stagnation and indigestible food.

33. Ascites

Recipe 1: Garlic cloves 250 g, one watermelon, and *sharen* (砂 仁 , Grains of Paradise) 120 g.

Prescription: After opening the watermelon at one end and removing the pulp, the garlic and *sharen* are placed in the melon with the opening covered by the original piece of rind. Mud is applied all over the melon and sundried, then the watermelon is baked over a woodfire. The dry melon rind is then ground into a powder for oral administration with water, 1.5 g, twice a day. After the ascites is eliminated, salt and watermelon are not to be eaten.

Explanation: This preparation can clear heat and increase the discharge of urine for treating ascites due to various causes such as cirrhosis of the liver, nutritional edema, and edema due to spleen deficiency.

Recipe 2: Two bulbs of garlic with skin peeled, mung beans 400 g, and a small amount of sugar.

Prescription: The mung beans are soaked in water for 4 hours and boiled with garlic over a low flame until the beans are very soft for 3 times of oral administration a day, after adding some sugar. This should be repeated for 7 successive days as a therapeutic course. This treatment should be stopped if it is ineffective after 2 therapeutic courses. Salt and spicy foods are prohibited during this course of treatment.

Explanation: This recipe can clear heat, increase the discharge of urine and relieve toxicity for treating ascites due to schistosomiasis in the late stages.

Recipe 3: A blank fish (a little more than 400 g) and an adequate amount of single-clove garlic.

Prescription: After the fish is killed and cleaned, the body cavity is filled with garlic and the body surface is covered with mud and baked over a charcoal fire for oral administration.

Explanation: This method can nourish the spleen, promote urination, resolve edema, and relieve toxicity in treating edema and ascites. A carp, with the scales, may be substituted for the blank fish.

34. Malaria

Recipe 1: One bulb of single-clove garlic and 10 peach pits.

Prescription: The garlic and peach pits are boiled and then taken in one dose.

Explanation: Malaria, caused by plasmodia and transmitted by the anopheline mosquito, usually occurs in summer and can be divided into tertian malaria, quartan malaria, and pernicious malaria. Patients may suffer from paroxysmal attacks of chills, high fever, headache, sweating, and splenomegaly.

Recipe 2: An adequate amount of dried ginger.

Prescription: Dried ginger is ground into black powder for oral administration with warm wine before the onset of paroxysmal attack of chills and high fever.

Explanation: This is an effective method for treating malaria.

Recipe 3: An adequate amount of single-clove garlic and yellow lead.

Prescription: The garlic and yellow lead are pounded together to prepare pills the size of longan. The pills are sundried and stored for use. In the morning before the onset of paraxysmal attacks, one pill is taken with water.

Explanation: This perparation is used to treat malaria with periodic attacks of chills and high fever.

Recipe 4: Fresh ginger 3 g and ginseng 3 g.

Prescription: These herbs are boiled in 200 ml water to prepare a decoction of 100 ml and stored overnight. Before oral administration, the decoction should be boiled again.

Explanation: This recipe is used to treat malaria due to retention of phlegm in the spleen with episodes of chills and fever, slight abdominal distention, cold limbs, and soft pulse.

Recipe 5: Fresh ginger 9 g and preserved fine tea leaves 9 g.

Prescription: A concentrated decoction or a decoction of these herbs, slightly fried, is prepared for oral administration.

Explanation: This recipe is used in treating dysentery with pus and blood in stool, and malaria with episodes of chills and fever.

Recipe 6: Fresh ginger with skin 120 g.

Prescription: The ginger is pounded to prepare juice. After storing overnight, cold ginger juice of 50 ml is taken before breakfast.

Explanation: This method is used to treat malaria due to retention of phlegm in the spleen and stomach with repeated episodes of chills and fever.

35. Constipation

Recipe 1: One stalk of green onion the thickness of the little finger and a small amount of honey.

Prescription: The green onion is dipped in honey and then inserted into the anus to a depth of 5-6 cm, then pulled out and inserted again 2-3 times. The stools may pass 20 minutes after treatment.

Explanation: This method can lubricate the intestines to facilitate bowel movement. This preparation is not for oral administration.

Recipe 2: Three green onion stalks and 7 pieces of *dandouchi* (淡 豆 豉, Medicated Soybean).

Prescription: The cleaned green onion is pounded with *dandouchi* to prepare a paste for application over the umbilicus then covered with cloth.

Explanation: This method can clear heat, moisten aridity in the intestines, and promote the passage of stools in treating constipation caused by heat pathogen.

Recipe 3: Green onion 120 g.

Prescription: A paste of green onion is made and applied over the umbilical region and covered with a hot towel or hot-water bag.

Explanation: This method is useful for treating constipation, and is especially effective for women who have recently given birth.

Recipe 4: Green onion stalks 2,000 g.

Prescription: The green onion is cut into slivers and fried with vinegar. The hot fried onion is divided into 2 portions and wrapped in 2 bags for hot compresses applied alternately over the umbilicus.

Explanation: In general, the stool will pass 6 hours after treatment.

Recipe 5: Green onion 16 g, fresh ginger 6 g, radish juice 12 g, and table salt 20 g.

Prescription: These herbs are mixed together and fried for application of a hot compress over the umbilicus.

Explanation: This method can be used to treat constipation due to an accumulation of heat in the stomach and intestines with stagnation of qi.

Recipe 6: Ginger about one inch long with the thickness of a thumb.

Prescription: The ginger is wrapped in paper and baked over fire. The hot ginger is inserted into the anus after being dipped in sesame oil. The stool may be passed half a day to one day later.

Explanation: This method is useful for treating constipation of the deficient type in aged people.

Recipe 7: One bulb of single-clove garlic.

Prescription: After peeling the skin, the garlic is baked over fire and the hot garlic wrapped in silk floss is inserted into the anus.

Explanation: This method is used to treat stubborn constipation.

Recipe 8: Fresh ginger 15 g, a whole green onion, a small pinch of salt, and *dandouchi* (淡 豆 豉, Medicated Soybean) 30 grains.

Prescription: These herbs are pounded and mixed together, and after baking over a fire, the hot paste is applied into the umbilicus and secured by a bandage. After the warmth penetrating through the body subsides, the paste may be replaced by a new piece of hot paste.

Explanation: This method is used to treat retention of urine and stool in aged people.

Recipe 9: A handful of green onion, some musk and salt.

Prescription: The musk is put into the umbilicus and covered with salt. The green onion is tied over a segment 1 cm in length. After both ends of green onion are cut away, the bundle of short segments of green onion is put over the umbilicus and ironed with a hot water container made of tin.

Explanation: This method is used to treat retention of urine and stool in critical patients.

36. Hematochezia (Anal Bleeding)

Recipe 1: Fresh ginger 15 g and *aiye* (艾 叶, Leaf of Mugwort) 15 g.

Prescription: One cup of a concentrated decoction of these herbs is taken.

Explanation: The mugwort can warm the meridians and stop

bleeding, and the fresh ginger can expel cold pathogen for treating anal bleeding after bowel movements of the deficient cold type.

Recipe 2: Five bowls of vinegar and three bowls of red beans.
Prescription: After boiling in vinegar and dried, the red beans are ground to prepare a powder for oral administration in a dosage of 5 g.
Explanation: This preparation is used to treat anal bleeding from hemorrhoids.

Recipe 3: Three green onion stalks.
Prescription: A decoction of green onion is made and used to steam and wash the anus.
Explanation: This method is used to treat anal bleeding from hemorrhoids.

Recipe 4: Fresh ginger 10 g and *aiye* (艾 叶, Leaf of Mugwort) 10 g.
Prescription: The decoction is made by these ingredients and then taken.
Explanation: Anal bleeding with or without stool, before or after defecation, is all called hematochezia.

37. Prolapse of Anus

Recipe: Green onion with red scales and Chinese chives.
Prescription: A decoction of these plants with roots, *dafengzi* (大 风 子, Chaulmoogra) and *fangfeng* (防 风, Saposhniko-via Root) is used to wash the perineal region.
Explanation: This recipe can raise kidney yang and restore a prolapsed anus.

38. Cerebral Apoplexy (Stroke)

Recipe 1: Fresh ginger 3 g, *jingjie* (荆 芥, Schizonepeta) 30 g, *xuanfuhua* (旋 复 花, Inula Flower) 20 g, and *niubangzi* (牛 蒡 子, Burdock Fruit) 20 g.
Prescription: A decoction of these ingredients is made and

orally administered, 3 times a day.

Explanation: This recipe is used to treat hemiplegia, deviation of mouth and eyes, and numbness of muscles and skin due to a depletion of qi and blood in meridians, and an invasion of wind pathogen to internal organs of the body; deficiency of liver and kidney yin and upward invasion of wind and yang pathogen; or accumulation of heat and phlegm pathogen in internal organs and an upward invasion of wind and phlegm pathogen.

Recipe 2: A lump of fresh ginger and a Chinese blister beetle.

Prescription: After the head is removed, the blister beetle is obliquely placed on the mandibular joint and covered with ginger paste for 3-4 hours, once a day.

Explanation: This method is used to treat deviation of the mouth and eyes caused by stroke.

Recipe 3: Two cloves of garlic.

Prescription: The garlic paste is applied on the gums in mouth.

Explanation: This method is used to treat aphasia by opening the orifices of the sense organs.

Recipe 4: Fresh ginger 30 g and one big fresh *fuzi* (附 子, Monkshood) cut into 8 slices.

Prescription: These herbs are boiled in 400 ml of water to prepare 100 ml of warm decoction for oral administration.

Explanation: This recipe can be used to treat strokes of any type with unconsciousness and excessive excretion of saliva.

Recipe 5: A handful of green onion stalks, with roots and a handful of cypress leaves.

Prescription: These herbs are ground to prepare a paste and then boiled in 60 ml of wine for oral administration.

Explanation: This recipe should be used to treat comatose stroke patients with lockjaw, aphasia, and excessive excretion of saliva to prevent disabling complications.

Recipe 6: Ginger juice 50 ml and sesame oil 100 ml.

Prescription: A mixture of these two ingredients is slowly administered to the stroke patient.

Explanation: This method is used to treat patients with aphasia due to stagnation of excessive phlegm.

Recipe 7: Chopped garlic 500 g and fried soybeans 1,000 g.

Prescription: The garlic and soybeans are boiled in 80 ml of water on a low flame to prepare a sticky paste for oral administration of 100-200 ml a day before meals.

Explanation: This preparation can nourish kidney qi for treating aged stroke patients with stagnation of toxic pathogen in the internal organs.

39. Facial Paralysis

Recipe 1: One bulb of garlic and fresh celery 50 g.

Prescription: A paste of these vegetables is applied to the normal side of the face once a day.

Explanation: This method is used to treat deviation of mouth and eyes until the deformity is corrected.

Recipe 2: Fresh ginger 15 g, almond 30 g and *xixin* (细 辛 , Wild Ginger) 6 g.

Prescription: A paste of these herbs is applied to the normal side of the face once a day.

Explanation: This method is used to treat deviation of mouth and eyes in stroke patients.

Recipe 3: Green onion stalks 30 g and fennel seedling 30 g.

Prescription: A paste of these vegetables is applied to the normal side of the face, once a day.

Explanation: This method is used to treat facial paralysis with deviation of the mouth and eyes.

Recipe 4: Fresh ginger 15 g, *baijiezi* (白 芥 子 , White Mustard Seed) 15 g, and honey 10 ml.

Prescription: A paste of these ingredients is applied to the normal side of the face, once a day.

Explanation: This paste can promote circulation of qi, release stagnation in the meridians, and stop pain in treating deviation of the mouth and eyes due to blockage of the meridians.

40. Insomnia

Recipe 1: Eight green onion stalks, 15 red dates, and sugar 5 g.

Prescription: These ingredients are boiled in two bowls of water to prepare a bowl of decoction for oral administration before going to bed.

Explanation: This decoction is used to treat insomnia in neurasthenia patients. It may produce a better effect if the patients soak their feet in hot water for a long time before going to bed.

Recipe 2: Green onion stalks 150 g.

Prescription: The green onion stalks are cut into small bits and put in a small dish beside the pillow at bedtime. The patient may then fall asleep peacefully.

Explanation: This method can relax the mind for treating insomnia due to neurasthenia.

Recipe 3: Seven green onion stalks and 20 red dates.

Prescription: A decoction of these ingredients is taken.

Explanation: This recipe can nourish the heart and relax the mind of weak and worried insomnia sufferers.

41. Intercostal Neuralgia

Recipe: Dried ginger 3 g, ginseng 3 g, and *baizhu* (白 术, Largehead Atractylodis) 3 g.

Prescription: A decoction of these herbs is orally administered, 3 times a day.

Explanation: This recipe is used to treat intercostal neuralgia in patients with severe pain, cold limbs, anxiety, and deep and slow pulse.

42. Sexual Neurosis

Recipe: An adequate amount of garlic.

Prescription: Three cloves of clean garlic are taken with or after meals.

Explanation: This method may produce a good effect if continued for a long time.

43. Lumbago

Recipe 1: Fresh ginger juice 120 g and gelatin 30 g.

Prescription: The ginger juice and gelatin are boiled to prepare a paste, and then spread over a piece of kraft paper for application over the painful area.

Explanation: This preparation can relieve muscle spasm, expel cold pathogen, and release blood stasis for treating lumbago.

Recipe 2: Dried ginger 6 g, *fuling* (茯 苓, Poria Coccus) 6 g, *gancao* (甘 草, Licorice) 3 g, and *baizhu* (白 术, Largehead Atratylodis) 3 g.

Prescription: A decoction of these herbs is orally administered before a meal.

Explanation: This recipe is used to treat lumbago patients with heaviness and cold in the waist due to kidney deficiency and an attack of damp pathogen. The patient has no desire to drink water, but urination is normal.

Recipe 3: An adequate amount of fresh ginger and mustard.

Prescription: A powder of these two ingredients is mixed with wine to prepare a paste for application over the affected area.

Explanation: This preparation is used to treat pain and distension of the back and waist.

Recipe 4: Fresh ginger 10 g, *mugua* (木 瓜, Flowering Quince Fruit) 30 g, and *cheqianzi* (车 前 子, Plantain Seed in a cloth bag) 30 g.

Prescription: A decoction of these herbs is orally administered, twice a day.

Explanation: This recipe is used to treat lumbago of rheumatism.

Recipe 5: Fresh ginger 100 g and *chunshuye* (椿 树 叶, Leaves of Tree of Heaven) 100 g.

Prescription: A paste of these two ingredients is applied on the back, once a day.

Explanation: This method is used to treat chronic lumbago caused by cold and damp pathogens.

44. Convulsions

Recipe: Ginger juice 6 g and pig bone 600 g.

Prescription: These ingredients are boiled in water to prepare a soup of 150 ml, mixed with 25 ml of wine for 3 oral administrations.

Explanation: This soup is used to treat repeated attacks of convulsions with pain in the fingers and the patient unable to stand for long because of weakness.

45. Beriberi

Recipe 1: Fresh garlic 20 cloves, fresh peanuts 250 g, and 6 chicken claws.

Prescription: These ingredients are boiled in water for oral administration until the edema is resolved.

Explanation: The peanuts contain cephalin, which is useful for treating intestinal obstructions and beriberi.

Recipe 2: Peanuts 200 g, red beans 200 g, garlic 200 g, and brown sugar 200 g.

Prescription: These ingredients are well boiled until softened for oral administration, once a day. This preparation may lose its therapeutic effect if salt is added to it.

Explanation: This preparation can be used to treat beriberi with edema of the foot, and ankle joint with some discomfort of the leg. Patients with edema spreading upward over the knee and thigh are very critical and should go to a hospital for emergency treatment.

Recipe 3: Dried ginger 4 g, *muxiang* (木 香 , Costus Root) 4 g, old wine 4 g, and plums 2 g.

Prescription: These herbs are boiled in 400 ml of water until 200 ml of decoction is obtained for oral administration, 3 times a day.

Explanation: This recipe is used to prevent heart disease from beriberi. At the same time, the patient should also take a large dose of vitamin B1.

Recipe 4: Garlic 60 g, ginger 30 g, *chenpi* (陈 皮 , Dried Tangerine Peel) 30 g, red beans 60 g, and one carp fish.

Prescription: After washing clean, the carp is well boiled with the other ingredients for oral administration.

Explanation: The occurrence and development of beriberi is closely related to the spleen and stomach, and the edema of beriberi can be resolved after the functions of the spleen and stomach are restored. The red beans and carp, supported by the tangerine peel can resolve edema.

Recipe 5: Green onion 100 g and radish seed 50 g.

Prescription: The ingredients are boiled in water for one hour to obtain a bowl of decoction for one oral administration.

Explanation: This is used in treating beriberi with edema and pain.

Recipe 6: One piece of green onion, fresh ginger 45 g, and *aiye* (艾 叶 , Leaf of Mugwort) 60 g.

Prescription: After pounding, the paste of green onion and ginger is mixed with the mugwort and wrapped in a cloth bag. After soaking in hot liquor, it is used to rub the affected area until the pain is relieved.

Explanation: This method is used to relieve pain in both feet and legs caused by damp pathogen.

46. Night Sweating

Recipe: One bulb of garlic and one snakegourd fruit.

Prescription: The snakegourd fruit is fried with garlic paste for oral administration, 1-2 times a day.

Explanation: This method can nourish yin and clear heat for treating night sweating due to yin deficiency.

47. Leprosy

Recipe: Green onion stalks 30 g, garlic 50 g, and chili 20 g.

Prescription: These ingredients are pounded together to prepare a paste for application over the lesions areas.

Explanation: Leprosy is a chronic infectious disease caused by bacillus leprae involving the skin and periperal nerves. Sometimes, deep tissue and internal organs may also be injured. Leprosy sufferers are the only source of infection.

48. Nephritis

Recipe 1: One bulb of garlic and 50 castor beans.

Prescription: A paste of these herbs is applied to the soles and changed once every 12 hours until a diuretic and edema-resolving effect is produced.

Explanation: Glomerulonephritis is an allergic disease following an infection of hemolytic streptococcus caused by an attack of cold weather, chronic fatigue, and a lowering of body resistance.

Recipe 2: Fresh ginger 10 g and *qianniuzi* (牵 牛 子, Pharbitis Seed) 12 g.

Prescription: A decoction of these two herbs is orally administered.

Explanation: This recipe is used to treat nephritis edema, but it is contraindicated for weak patients.

Recipe 3: Several cloves of garlic and one watermelon.

Prescription: The watermelon is opened at one end with the pulp and seeds all removed. The empty cavity is filled with garlic, the opening is closed with the original piece of rind and the whole melon is covered with mud and baked in burning chaff. After the mud is removed, the baked watermelon with garlic is ground to prepare a powder for oral administration of 5 g, twice a day.

Explanation: This preparation can promote the discharge of urine for treating edema in chronic nephritis patients.

Recipe 4: Garlic 50 g and one wild duck.

Prescription: After the feathers and viscera are removed and the duck is washed clean, the garlic is put into the body cavity and boiled until the duck meat is well-done. The duck meat and soup is taken for three successive days. This treatment should be continued until several ducks are eaten.

Explanation: This preparation can nourish spleen and stomach qi and clean blocked orifices to discharge urine. This is a useful treatment for chronic nephritis with edema.

Recipe 5: An adequate amount of garlic and one carp.

Prescription: After the scales and viscera are removed and the fish is well washed, the garlic bits are put into the body cavity and the fish is wrapped in lotus leaf and baked in burning chaff until the fish meat is well-done for oral administration.

Explanation: This preparation can produce a warming and tonic effect to promote the discharge of water and relieve nausea and vomiting in patients with chronic nephritis.

Recipe 6: Two bulbs of garlic and watermelon pulp 25 g.

Prescription: The garlic cloves are put on the melon pulp and steamed for two oral administrations a day.

Explanation: This method is used chiefly to treat glomerulonephritis, and as a supplemental treatment also useful for other kidney diseases.

49. Dribbling Urination

Recipe 1: One bulb of garlic.

Prescription: The garlic is wrapped in paper and baked.

After exposure overnight, the baked garlic is taken before breakfast with cool water.

Explanation: The garlic has a pungent odor and a warm nature, so it is useful for treating dribbling urination of the deficient-cold type.

Recipe 2: An adequate amount of green onion stalks and salt.

Prescription: The green onion stalks and salt are fried for application of a hot compress over the umbilicus and abdomen.

Explanation: The green onion stalks can promote circulation of yang and expel cold pathogen for treating impaired urination due to dysfunction of the urinary bladder.

Recipe 3: An adequate amount of garlic and *dandouchi* (淡豆豉, Medicated Soybean).

Prescription: A steamed paste of these ingredients is used to prepare small pills for oral administration, 30-40 pills each time, three times a day for 3 days to control dribbling urination.

Explanation: This method is used to treat dribbling urination of various types.

50. Retention of Urine

Recipe 1: One bulb of single-clove garlic, 20 Cape Jasmine (Fructus Gardeniae) and some salt.

Prescription: These herbs are ground to prepare powder which is mixed with water to form a paste applied over the umbilicus.

Explanation: This method is used to treat retention of urine with distention and pain below the umbilicus.

Recipe 2: Green onion 15 g and alum 9 g.

Prescription: A paste of these ingredients is applied to the umbilicus.

Explanation: The retention of urine is a disease of the urinary bladder.

Recipe 3: Green onion 500 g and a small amount of musk.

Prescription: A paste of green onion is fried hot and mixed

with musk for application over the umbilicus. A piece of hot new paste is applied when the original paste become cool.

Explanation: This method is used to treat retention of urine with distention of the lower abdomen.

Recipe 4: Fresh ginger 9 g and *qianniuzi* (牵 牛 子, Pharbitis Seeds) 12 g.

Prescription: A decoction of these ingredients is prepared for oral administration.

Explanation: Both herbs can warm and nourish kidney yang, clear heat, eliminate dampness and resolve edema for treating retention of urine.

Recipe 5: One bulb of single-clove garlic, 30 Cape Jasmine and some salt.

Prescription: The paste of these herbs is spread over paper and then applied to the umbilicus for a long time to promote discharge of urine.

Explanation: This recipe can clear heat, relieve toxicity and promote discharge of urine for treating urine retention due to an accumulation of heat and damp pathogens in the body.

Recipe 6: Green onion stalks 12 g and some salt.

Prescription: The umbilicus is filled with salt and covered with a green onion paste. Then moxibustion is applied with the burned moxa cone placed on the green onion paste until the burning sensation on the abdominal wall is intolerable and the urine is discharged.

Explanation: This method can warm the spleen and stomach, nourish qi, and promote discharge of urine and stool in treating retention of urine caused by an attack of wind pathogen after child birth in women.

Recipe 7: Five bulbs of garlic, 4 large snails, and *cheqianzi* (车 前 子, Plantain Seed) 15 g.

Prescription: The ingredients are pounded to make cakes for application to the umbilicus fixed by a bandage until the urine is discharged.

Explanation: This method can eliminate dampness and resolve swelling for treating ascites, edema, and retention of urine.

Recipe 8: An adequate amount of green onion stalks and *shanglu* (商 陆 , Poke Root).
Prescription: A mixed powder of these herbs is placed into the umbilicus.
Explanation: This method can promote discharge of water and resolve edema to treat retention of urine.

Recipe 9: Fifty dry stems of garlic, 8 roots of green onion, and 8 outer leaves of Chinese cabbage.
Prescription: The ingredients are boiled in water for steaming and washing the perineal region until sweating is induced in this region and urine is discharged.
Explanation: This method can clear heat, promote discharge of urine, and relieve toxicity to treat dribbling urination with distention and pain in lower abdomen.

Recipe 10: An equal amount of green onion stalks and snail meat.
Prescription: A hot paste of these ingredients is applied to Guanyuan (CV 4) acupoint. For patients with distention and pain in lower abdomen the slivers of stalks of greeen onion are fried and wrapped in a gauze bag for hot ironing over the lower abdomen. The urine may be discharged after the hot sensation penetrates the abdominal wall.
Explanation: Guanyuan is an acupoint 3 *cun* (unit of length for locating acupoints) below the umbilicus.

Recipe 11: Green onion with roots 100 g and table salt 15 g.
Prescription: A hot paste of these ingredients is applied to the umbilical region.
Explanation: A paste applied over the abdomen should not be very hot to avoid a burn injury to the skin.

51. Incontinence of Urine

Recipe: Dried ginger 2 g and *gancao* (甘 草 , Licorice) 4 g.

Prescription: The herbs are boiled in 200 ml of water to prepare 100 ml of decoction for oral administration, 2 times a day.

Explanation: This recipe is used to treat frequent urination and incontinence of urine in weak aged people. According to traditional Chinese medical theory, incontinence of urine is due to a deficiency of kidney qi.

52. Emission

Recipe: Dried ginger 30 g, *chishizhi* (赤 石 脂, Red Halloysite) 30 g, and pepper 15 g.

Prescription: A powder of these herbs is used to prepare pills, with vinegar and wheat flour, the size of the seeds of the parasol tree, for oral administration of 5-7 pills with rice gruel.

Explanation: This recipe is used to treat male patients with diarrhea and emission.

53. Impotence

Recipe 1: Three fresh thick leaves of green onion (with mucus) and 7 fresh shelled sea shrimp.

Prescription: The shrimp meat is put into the leaves of green onion. After sundrying, they are ground into powder for oral administration with tea twice a day.

Explanation: This preparation can nourish the kidney, enrich essence, and promote the circulation of yang and qi to treat impotence and premature ejaculation of semen.

Recipe 2: A lump of ripe ginger.

Prescription: The hot roasted ginger with skin peeled is inserted into the anus to stimulate erection of the penis.

Explanation: This method can relieve exterior syndrome and warm the spleen and stomach for treating poor erection of the penis.

54. Bi-Syndrome (Arthritis)

Recipe 1: An adequate amount of fresh ginger, sulfur, and

aiye (艾 叶, Mugwort Leaf).

Prescription: A hot baked powder of these herbs is applied to the affected areas.

Explanation: Bi-syndrome is a group of diseases with pain, soreness, numbness and swelling of the ligaments, muscle, bone and joints and limitation of movement due to impaired qi and blood circulation caused by an attack of wind, cold, and damp pathogens.

Recipe 2: Fresh ginger juice 90 g and green onion juice 90 g.

Prescription: A mixture of these juices is boiled with gum 150 g for application after spreading over a piece of silk.

Explanation: This method is used to treat the pain of Bi-syndrome due to various causes.

Recipe 3: Ginger juice 25 g, green onion juice 25 g, vinegar 25 g, wheat flour 50 g, and ox skin glue 25 g.

Prescription: A paste made of these ingredients is applied over the affected area to control pain.

Explanation: This preparation is useful for treating acute gout.

Recipe 4: Equal amounts of fresh ginger and old wheat.

Prescription: A hot fried ginger paste is applied to the knee and wrapped with a silk bandage for two nights, and then the hot fried granules of wheat are applied to the knee.

Explanation: This method is used to treat swollen knee joints.

Recipe 5: Single-clove garlic 200 g, fresh ginger 200 g, green onion 200 g, yellow lead 400 g, and one entire sloughed snake skin.

Prescription: These ingredients (except the yellow lead) are fried in oil and then mixed with the yellow lead after the dregs are removed to prepare a paste for application to the painful area.

Explanation: In this recipe, green onion and ginger can expel cold pathogen and promote circulation of yang, and garlic can relieve swelling and pain, and the snake skin is useful for treating rheumatic pain in the bones and joints.

Recipe 6: An adequate amount of fresh ginger and one green onion stalks.

Prescription: The ginger and green onion are pounded and mixed with wheat flour to prepare a paste. After frying, the hot paste is applied over the affected area.

Explanation: This method is used to treat the inversion of arms and legs.

Recipe 7: Fresh ginger 10 g, stalk of green onion 60 g, peeled dried towel gourd 20 g, and *zuandifeng* (钻 地 风 , Radix Kadsurae Coccinae) 20 g.

Prescription: These herbs are pounded to prepare a paste for application over the affected area.

Explanation: This method is used to treat severe pain of the shoulder joints, which can be relieved by heat and exacerbated by cold.

Recipe 8: An adequate amount of fresh ginger, green onion, and fresh *aiye* (艾 叶, Leaf of Mugwort).

Prescription: The ingredients are pounded and fried with wine and then put in a cloth bag for application of a hot compress to the painful area.

Explanation: This method is used to treat pain and cold of the knee and foot.

Recipe 9: Equal amounts of fresh ginger and stalk of green onion.

Prescription: The bits of ginger and green onion are fried and put in a cloth bag for application of a hot compress, 3 times a day. After the bag is cool, it is replaced by a new hot bag.

Explanation: This method is used to treat chronic rheumatic arthritis which is a Bi-syndrome caused by cold pathogen or derived from a Bi-syndrome caused by wind pathogen.

Recipe 10: Equal amounts of wheat flour and ginger paste

(accounting for 10-20 percent of the total weight), and a taro.

Prescription: The peeled taro is ground into a paste and then thoroughly mixed with wheat flour and ginger paste for application.

Explanation: This method is used to treat pain of shoulder and wrist joints together with the practice of functional exercise by the patients.

Recipe 11: An adequate amount of large garlic and several moxa cones.

Prescription: The garlic is cut into slices each 2 mm thick and placed on the tender spot. The moxa cone is placed on the garlic slices for application of moxibustion until the garlic slices turn grey in color. During the first treatment, the garlic slices may be changed 3 times, and in the following treatments the number of garlic slices used for moxibustion may be gradually increased. This treatment is applied twice a day.

Explanation: This method is used to treat neuralgia caused by rheumatism of the muscles.

55. Rheumatoid Arthritis

Recipe 1: Roots of green onion 100 g, garlic cloves 100 g, and pepper 60 g.

Prescription: A hot decoction of these ingredients is used to steam and wash the sore spot, 3-4 times a day. One mixture of the above herbs can be used for 5 days.

Explanation: This method is used to treat rheumatoid arthritis or as a supplemental therapy for this ailment.

Recipe 2: Roots of green onion 15 g, fresh ginger 3 slices, black plum 10 g, and 10 red dates.

Prescription: A decoction of these ingredients is taken, 1-2 times a day.

Explanation: This recipe can eliminate wind pathogen and control pain in treating rheumatic arthritis.

56. Acute Arthritis

Recipe: Green onion stalks 50 g and mature vinegar 1,000 g.

Prescription: The vinegar is boiled until half of its original volume is left, and then boiled again with the slivers of green onion for a while. After filtering, a piece of cloth soaked with the hot vinegar is applied twice a day.

Explanation: This method can induce sweating and expel superficial pathogen to treat acute arthritis with pain and swelling.

57. Edema

Recipe 1: An adequate amount of ginger and pepper and a duck.

Prescription: After removing the duck feathers and viscera, its abdominal cavity is filled with ginger, pepper, and 500 g of rice. After the abdominal wall is sutured, the duck is steamed until the meat is well-done for oral administration.

Explanation: This preparation can produce good results in treating edema and abdominal distention.

Recipe 2: One bulb of garlic, fresh ginger 3 g, red beans 30 g, and one piece of *shanglu* (商 陆 , Poke Root) cut into slivers.

Prescription: These herbs are boiled until the red beans are softened for thorough chewing and swallowing after the other ingredients are removed. The bean gruel is completely eaten to resolve edema.

Explanation: This method can resolve edema due to various causes.

Recipe 3: Green onion stalks 500 g, fresh ginger 500 g, and white turnip 1,000 g.

Prescription: These vegetables are pounded to make a paste and fried in a pot for application of a hot compress to the umbilicus, Guanyuan (CV 4) and Pishu (BL 20) acupoints, after being put into two bags and used alternately.

Explanation: The Guanyuan acupoint lies 3 cun (unit of

length for locating acupoints) below the umbilicus, and the Pishu acupoint lies below the 11th thoracic vertebra and 1.5 cun beside the posterior median line.

Recipe 4: Garlic 30 g and *shanglu* (商 陆, Poke Root) 3 g.
Prescription: These herbs are boiled with meat for oral administration with sugar.
Explanation: This is a good method for treating edema, but salt is prohibited during treatment.

Recipe 5: Ginger peel 25 g, root of dandelion 50 g, and overgrown wax gourd skin 100 g.
Prescription: A decoction of these ingredients is prepared for oral administration.
Explanation: This recipe is used to treat patients with acute general edema, anuria, thirst, and rapid pulse. Salt is prohibitated for one week.

Recipe 6: An adequate amount of garlic cloves and large snails.
Prescription: The snail meat is pounded with garlic to prepare a paste for application to an area 3 fingers wide below the umbilicus (not into the umbilicus) and over the soles of both feet, wrapped in a bandage.
Explanation: This method can clear heat, eliminate dampness, promote discharge of urine, relieve toxicity and resolve edema in treating general edema, anuria, and abdominal distention.

58. Heat Stroke

Recipe 1: An adequate amount of fresh ginger or garlic.
Prescription: The ginger or garlic is swallowed with hot water after thorough chewing, and a hot, wet cloth compress is applied at Qihai (CV 6) acupoint, then the patient may regain consciousness.
Explanation: This method is used to treat collapsed patients who have suddenly fallen and are incontinent of urine with

spontaneous sweating, chills and fever, and cold limbs. Cold water should not be used for drinking or bathing the patients because it may cause sudden death.

Recipe 2: An adequate amount of fresh ginger, garlic, and Chinese chives.

Prescription: After washing and peeling, these ingredients are pounded to produce a juice for oral administration.

Explanation: This juice can relieve exterior syndrome, warm the spleen and stomach, and stimulate nerve functions in treating victims of heat stroke who have collapsed and are unconscious.

Recipe 3: Two bulbs of garlic.

Prescription: A garlic paste is fed to the patient with water.

Explanation: This method is used to treat collapsed heat stroke victims.

Recipe 4: Two drops of ginger juice, brown sugar 12 g, mung beans 20 g, and lotus leaf 30 g.

Prescription: A decoction of these ingredients is orally administered several times a day.

Explanation: This recipe is used to prevent heat stroke.

59. Toxicity

Recipe 1: Garlic 30 g, mung bean 60 g, *cheqiancao* (车 前 草, Plantain) 10 g, and *yuxingcao* (鱼 腥 草, Houttuymia) 30 g.

Prescription: A decoction of these herbs is orally administered several times a day.

Explanation: This recipe is used to treat food poisoning causing a mild and slow toxic reaction.

Recipe 2: Garlic 1.5 g.

Prescription: The garlic is taken once a day for 3 months.

Explanation: The garlic can produce a strong detoxifying effect to prevent and treat lead poisoning.

Recipe 3: Garlic and realgar in a ratio of 2:1 by weight.

Prescription: The garlic and realgar are soaked in alcohol and bottled for use.

Explanation: This preparation is used to treat toxicity due to insect bites.

Recipe 4: Fresh ginger 50 g, *zisuye* (紫 苏 叶, Leaf of Perilla) 50 g, and an adequate amount of brown sugar.

Prescription: A decoction of these herbs is taken, twice a day.

Explanation: This is a good method for treating food poisoning from fish and crab.

Recipe 5: Fresh ginger 10 g.

Prescription: The cold ginger decoction is orally administered.

Explanation: This decoction is used particularly for intoxication of *banxia* (半 夏, Ternate Pinellia). This treatment should be continued for as longer as it takes to relieve toxicity.

Recipe 6: Fresh ginger 10 g, bean milk 250 ml, and crystal sugar 30 g.

Prescription: The ginger and sugar are boiled in bean milk for oral administration, 1-2 times a day.

Explanation: This method is used to treat alcohol intoxication.

Recipe 7: Green onion stalks 15 g and *douchi* (豆 豉, Medicated Soybean) 15 g.

Prescription: The ingredients are boiled in 300 ml of water until 200 ml of decoction is obtained for oral administration to dispel the effect of alcohol.

Explanation: This recipe is used to treat alcohol poisoning.

Recipe 8: Baked ginger filed into fine bits 30 g and *huanglian* (黄 连, Goldthread) slightly fried 30 g.

Prescription: A powder of these herbs is taken.

Explanation: This preparation is used to treat Croton poisoning with uncontrollable diarrhea.

Recipe 9: Fresh ginger 3 slices and clove powder 5 g.

Prescription: These herbs are boiled in 100 ml of water to prepare a warm decoction of 20 ml for oral administration.

Explanation: This is a good method for treating food poisoning from crab.

60. Epidemic Encephalitis B

Recipe 1: One bulb of garlic, mung beans 15 g and raw *gancao* (甘 草 , Licorice) 3 g.

Prescription: A decoction of these herbs is taken, 1-2 times a day.

Explanation: The garlic can relieve toxicity, the mung beans can clear heat and relieve toxicity, and *gancao* can modulate the effect of other herbs and relieve toxicity.

Recipe 2: Garlic clove 60 g and wild chrysanthemum 30 g.

Prescription: A concentrated decoction of these herbs is used for gargling.

Explanation: This recipe can clear heat and relieve toxicity. The fresh garlic may be taken and then rinsed with salt water several times a day to prevent encephalitis.

61. Shock

Recipe: Fresh ginger juice one cup, and alum 6 g.

Prescription: The alum is dissolved in water and drunk by the patient with ginger juice.

Explanation: This recipe can expel wind pathogen and warm the spleen and stomach for treating stroke, shock, and coma.

62. Cancer

Recipe 1: An adequate amount of garlic and one live crucian carp.

Prescription: The garlic slices are placed into the abdominal cavity of the carp after its scales and viscera have been removed. The fish is wrapped with paper and covered with mud and then baked over a fire so its therapeutic effect is not destroyed. After the mud is removed, the charcoal of fish is ground to prepare powder (or pills) for oral administration of 5 g, 2-3 times a day with rice gruel.

Explanation: This preparation can adjust stomach functions and transport qi downward to treat cancer of the esophagus and stomach at the early stages with gastrointestinal tract bleeding and vomiting.

Recipe 2: Fresh garlic 250 g and two and a half bottles of liquor.

Prescription: The garlic is completely immersed and soaked in liquor for more than one year. When ready, a small cup of garlic liquor is drunk before meals, twice a day.

Explanation: This method is used particularly for cancer of the stomach. It may also be used to treat other cancers on a trial basis.

63. Diabetes Mellitus

Recipe 1: Small bits of dried ginger and the bile of three crucian carp gallbladders.

Prescription: Five pills made of these ingredients are taken with rice gruel.

Explanation: This preparation can clear heat, suppress hyperactivity of the liver, eliminate dampness, and adjust the spleen and stomach functions in treating diabetes mellitus.

Recipe 2: Fresh ginger 2 slices, salt 4.5 g, and green tea 6 g.

Prescription: Five liters of tea is made with these ingredients for constant drinking.

Explanation: This method can clear heat and moisten dryness in the body for treating diabetes with thirst, irritability, and excessive urination.

Recipe 3: Fresh green onion 100 g and a small amount of plant oil.

Prescription: After washing and soaking in boiled water, the green onion is cut into fine slivers and mixed with plant oil as a vegetable salad taken with meal, twice a day.

Explanation: This salad can treat diabetes with symptoms of thirst, excessive urination, overeating, and pathological leanness.

Recipe 4: An adequate amount of green onion, fresh ginger, Chinese yam, and one pig tripe.

Prescription: The slivers of pig tripe and slices of Chinese yam are fried with chopped green onion and ginger to prepare a dish for oral administration with meals twice a day.

Explanation: The preparation is useful for treating excessive urination in diabetic patients.

Chapter 3
SURGICAL CONDITIONS

1. Boils

Recipe 1: Fresh garlic and vinegar.

Prescription: Garlic paste is wrapped in sterilized gauze and squeezed to prepare juice. The mixture of garlic juice and vinegar is boiled on a low fire to prepare a paste for application over the boil once a day for 3 to 7 days.

Explanation: This method may produce better results in treating boils before suppuration, but it is also useful afterwards.

Recipe 2: An adequate amount of whole green onions.

Prescription: The green onion is pounded in a stone mortar to prepare a paste with vinegar for application to the boils.

Explanation: This method may produce good results in treating boils before suppuration, and can also promote the drainage of pus after suppuration.

Recipe 3: Seven stalks of green onion and an adequate amount of honey.

Prescription: These ingredients are pounded in a stone mortar to prepare a paste for application to the boils.

Explanation: This method is usually used in the early stages of boil growth. It must not be taken orally.

Recipe 4: Two bulbs of single-clove garlic and an adequate amount of sesame oil.

Prescription: A thick layer of garlic paste mixed with sesame oil is applied to the boil, and replaced by new soft paste when the original paste becomes dry.

Explanation: The garlic can kill pyogenic bacteria and resolve pustules in the common boil.

Recipe 5: An adequate amount of fresh ginger and potatoes.

Prescription: The potatoes and ginger are pounded in a ratio of 3:1 to prepare a paste for external application.

Explanation: This method is used to treat boils or furuncle. The furuncle is an acute pyogenic infection of a single hair follicle and sebaceous gland.

Recipe 6: Seven stalks of green onion and alum powder 9 g.

Prescription: A paste of these ingredients is divided into 7 portions. After taking one portion with 100 ml of hot wine, the patient lies in bed covered with a thick blanket, and after drinking green onion soup 600 ml to induce sweating, the blanket may be removed. The boil may be quickly cured.

Explanation: This method is useful for treating furuncles and other pyogenic infections in the early stages before pus forms.

Recipe 7: An adequate amount of green onion stored over winter, and raw honey.

Prescription: The skin surrounding the boil is pricked with a bamboo needle. Then a paste of these ingredients is applied over the lesion and covered with a piece of silk. Hot vinegar is used to wash the lesion. This paste must not be taken orally.

Explanation: This method can expel toxic pathogen in treating boils.

Recipe 8: An adequate amount of stewed green onion stalks and alum 30 g.

Prescription: These herbs are pounded to prepare a paste for making pills. After drying, 7.5 g of pills is administered orally with hot wine.

Explanation: These pills are used to treat various skin sores.

Recipe 9: Garlic 60 g and *wuzhuyu* (吴茱萸 , Evodia) 30 g.

Prescription: A powder of these herbs is applied to the boil,

3 times a day.

Explanation: This powder is used to treat stubborn ulcers and swellings.

Recipe 10: An adequate amount of green onion stalks, twig of pagoda tree and *wasong* (瓦 松, Stonecrop).

Prescription: Stonecrop, dried in shadow, is ground into powder. After washing the lesion with a decoction of green onion and twig of pagoda tree, the dry powder of Stonecrop is applied. It is most effective in an open wound.

Explanation: This method is useful for treating stubborn sores difficult to heal.

Recipe 11: Green onion stalks 500 g, purslane 500 g, and lime 500 g.

Prescription: The ingredients are pounded to prepare a paste, and then ground to prepare a powder after the paste is dried in shadow. The powder is applied over the sore after the dead tissue is removed by application of a corrosive agent.

Explanation: This powder is used to treat chronic ulcers of the leg, furuncles, and carbuncles.

2. Carbuncles and Cellulitis

Recipe 1: Green onion stalks 150 g and two pig gallbladders.

Prescription: A paste of green onion is mixed with the pig bile for external application.

Explanation: This method is useful for treating all types of carbuncles and cellulitis.

Recipe 2: An adequate amount of green onion stalks, honey, and wheat flour.

Prescription: According to the size of the lesion, these three ingredients are pounded and heated for application to the affected area.

Explanation: This method is used to treat carbuncles, cellulitis, and other pyogenic skin infections without suppuration. This preparation must not be taken orally.

Recipe 3: Green onion 60 g, dried ginger 15 g, and cinnamon twig 30 g.

Prescription: The herbs are pounded and boiled with vinegar and wheat flour to prepare a paste for application all over the lesion for 7 days.

Explanation: This preparation is used to treat carbuncles on the back, breast cancer, and furuncles, but it is contraindicated for ruptured carbuncles.

3. Erysipelas

Recipe 1: Fresh ginger 9 g and a small amount of honey.

Prescription: The baked ginger is ground to fine bits and mixed with honey for application to the lesion.

Explanation: This method can expel wind and eliminate dampness pathogen to treat erysipelas due to an attack of wind-heat or damp-heat pathogen.

Recipe 2: An adequate amount of dried ginger bits.

Prescription: The dried ginger bits are mixed in honey for application to the lesion to produce a quick therapeutic effect.

Explanation: This method is used to treat multicolored erysipelas scattered over the body.

4. Tuberculosis of Cervical Lymph Nodes

Recipe: Five pieces of green onion and 8 scorpions.

Prescription: The scorpions and green onion are chopped to prepare stuffing for dumplings.

Explanation: The contents of the dumplings should not be disclosed to the patient since this knowledge may cause nausea due to a psychological reaction.

5. Traumatic Injuries

Recipe 1: An adequate amount of green onion.

Prescription: A fried hot paste of green onion is repeatedly applied over the lesion until the pain is relieved.

Explanation: This method can relieve blood stasis, stop bleeding, resolve swelling, and relieve toxicity in treating traumatic injury.

Recipe 2: An adequate amount of fresh ginger and green onion stalks.

Prescription: These ingredients are pounded and mixed with an adequate amount of wheat flour. After frying, the hot paste is used as a hot compress over the lesion.

Explanation: This method is used to treat various types of traumatic injuries, but should not be over used in treating open wounds.

Recipe 3: Three pieces of green onion and fresh ginger 30 g.

Prescription: The green onion and ginger are pounded to prepare a paste for external application, once a day.

Explanation: This method is particularly useful for treating wounds of the hand together with the application of antibiotics.

Recipe 4: One green onion with roots and an adequate amount of resin.

Prescription: The chopped green onion is fried with resin to prepare a paste for application over the painful and swollen area.

Explanation: This method can resolve swelling and relieve the pain of traumatic injury.

Recipe 5: Green onion stalks 20 g, ripe ginger 6 g, Chinese chives 20 g, and vine of towel gourd 20 g.

Prescription: These ingredients are pounded to prepare a paste for application over the wound.

Explanation: This method is used to treat painful injuries and strains of muscles and ligaments causing limited movement.

Recipe 6: A small amount of green onion.

Prescription: After roasted over a fire, the juice squeezed from the cut end of green onion is applied over the wound.

Explanation: The juice of roasted onion can resolve blood stasis and relieve pain in treating finger and toe injuries.

Recipe 7: An adequate amount of fresh ginger and taro with a small amount of wheat flour.

Prescription: After peeling the skin, the taro is cut and pounded to prepare a paste with ginger juice and wheat flour for application to the lesion after spreading over a piece of cloth the same size as the wound, twice a day. In winter, the paste should be warmed before application. It should be prepared right before application and used the same day.

Explanation: This paste is used to treat sprains of the waist. In addition, the application of this paste over the right lower abdomen in patients with acute appendicitis may reduce fever and blood cell count to normal.

Recipe 8: An adequate amount of garlic.

Prescription: Two or three drops of garlic juice is dropped into the nostrils, only one time.

Explanation: This method is used to treat fainting after traumatic injury, but it is contraindicated for comas following brain trauma.

Recipe 9: Fresh ginger 20 g and fresh fennel seedlings 60 g.

Prescription: These two plants are pounded to prepare a paste for application over the lesion, once a day.

Explanation: This method is used to treat acute sprain of the waist.

Recipe 10: One handful of green onion and 3-4 shed skins of cicada.

Prescription: These herbs are pounded to prepare a paste for application on the lesion once a day.

Explanation: This paste can effectively resolve swelling in treating traumatic injury.

6. Soft Tissue Injury

Recipe 1: An adequate amount of fresh ginger and green

onion stalks.

Prescription: The ingredients are pounded and mixed with wheat flour to prepare paste for a hot compress.

Explanation: This method may produce certain effects in treating traumatic injury to soft tissue with pain and swelling.

Recipe 2: An adequate amount of fresh ginger.

Prescription: The pounded ginger is fried with wheat flour for application over the lesion while it is hot.

Explanation: This method is used to treat hand and foot sprains.

7. Acute Sprain

Recipe 1: Two slices of fresh ginger and one spoonful of salt.

Prescription: Ginger is pounded and mixed with salt for application to the lesion, which is then wrapped with a bandage, once a day, for 2-3 days.

Explanation: This method is useful in treating acute sprains in the early stages with local swelling. The patient should start physical exercise after the swelling is resolved.

Recipe 2: An adequate amount of green onion stalks, ginger juice and yellow rice, and a small amount of wine.

Prescription: The hot fried green onion paste is applied first, then a mixture of wine and granules of yellow rice is applied to the lesion. The patient also may drink some good wine.

Explanation: This method is used to treat traumatic injuries of the waist with blood stasis and intolerable pain.

8. Calf Muscle Spasms

Recipe: One bulb of garlic.

Prescription: After peeling the skin, the garlic is used to rub the soles of the feet.

Explanation: This is an effective method for treating spasms of the calf muscles.

9. Animal and Insect Bites

Recipe 1: An adequate amount of garlic.

Prescription: Sliced garlic is applied to the painful area and the moxibustion with a burned moxa cone is applied over the sliced garlic.

Explanation: This method is used to treat snake, scorpion, and centipede bites.

Recipe 2: Two pieces of green onion and honey 30 g.

Prescription: A paste of green onion is mixed with honey for application to the lesion, once a day for 3 days.

Explanation: This paste can clear heat and relieve toxicity in treating poisonous snake, poisonous insect, centipede, bee, and scorpion bites. This paste must not be taken orally.

Recipe 3: One bulb of garlic and hot vinegar 40 g.

Prescription: A garlic paste is mixed with hot vinegar for application to the lesion.

Explanation: This method can be used for treating poisonous snake bites, but not for extremely poisonous snakes. Otherwise, the chance to save the life of critical patient bitten by a very poisonous snake may be lost.

10. Cut Wounds with Bleeding

Recipe 1: Five green onion stalks and white granulated sugar 2-3 g.

Prescription: These ingredients are pounded to prepare a paste for application over the wound which is then wrapped with a bandage.

Explanation: This method can heal wounds caused by knives and other sharp metal weapons.

Recipe 2: An adequate amount of green onion stalks.

Prescription: A hot paste of fried green onion is applied repeatedly over the wound.

Explanation: This method can quickly relieve the pain of wounds caused by metal weapons.

11. Tetanus

Recipe 1: Stored green onion stalks 500 g, black hyacinth beans 45 g, cotton seeds 90 g, and Chinese sorghum liquor 75 g.

Prescription:

(1) The cotton seeds are fried to a dark brown color, ground to fine bits, and strained to remove the skin.

(2) The green onion stalks are boiled in 4-5 bowls of water to prepare a soup.

(3) The black hyacinth beans are fried with white smoke and then blue smoke rising from the round-bottomed frying pan until 90 percent of the beans are burnt.

(4) A purple alcoholic fluid is obtained after the warm liquor is poured into the fried beans in the pan and filtered.

(5) This mixture of hyacinth bean liquor and cotton seed bits with an adequate amount of green onion soup is fed to the patient who is then covered with a heavy blanket to induce sweating, 1-2 times a day.

Explanation: This recipe can expel superficial pathogen, promote circulation of yang, and relieve toxicity in treating tetanus.

Recipe 2: One bulb of single-glove garlic, *weilingxian* (威 灵 仙, Chinese Clemetis) powder 15 g, and sesame oil 3 g.

Prescription: These herbs are pounded together for oral administration with hot wine to induce sweating.

Explanation: This recipe is used to treat injuries from metal weapons causing tetany.

12. Breast Ulceration

Recipe 1: An adequate amount of roots of green onion and a small amount of dried alum.

Prescription: The clean roots of green onion are pounded with dried alum to prepare pills, the size of soybeans for oral administration of 4 pills, 2-3 times a day to induce light sweating.

Explanation: This preparation can promote circulation of qi and blood and relieve swelling and blood stasis in treating ulcerations of the breast.

Recipe 2: Fresh green onion 250 g.

Prescription: After washing, cutting, pounding, squeezing, and heating, the hot juice of green onion is orally administered, once a day.

Explanation: The green onion juice can relieve toxicity, clear heat, and resolve swelling in treating breast ulcerations in women.

13. Breast Inflammation

Recipe 1: Small fresh green onions 100 g and deer horn powder 20 g.

Prescription: The juice of small green onions is mixed with an adequate amount of sweet wine for oral administration with 10 g of deer horn powder, twice a day.

Explanation: This recipe is used to treat inflammation in the early stages with stagnant milk.

Recipe 2: An adequate amount of fresh green onion stalks and raw *banxia* (半 夏, Ternate Pinellia).

Prescription: The green onion and *banxia* are pounded to prepare suppositories of a size suitable for application into the nostril on the side opposite the inflammation, for 20 minutes, twice a day.

Explanation: This method is used to treat acute inflammation in the early stages together with hot compresses and the suction of accumulated milk.

Recipe 3: Three pieces of green onion and an adequate amount of dandelion.

Prescription: The green onion and dandelion are pounded to prepare a paste for application over the lesion.

Explanation: This method can produce a good result in

treating simple inflammation.

14. Bone Fractures

Recipe: An adequate amount of green onion stalks and honey.

Prescription: The green onion is pounded with honey to prepare a paste for a thick layer of local application.

Explanation: This paste is used for skull fractures. It is for external application only and must not be orally administered.

15. Bone Tuberculosis

Recipe: A large amount of fresh or dried ginger.

Prescription: A ginger paste is boiled in water for over one hour for a hot towel compress over the lesion, twice a day.

Explanation: This treatment can produce a warming effect to relieve stagnant blood and stop pain in the tubercular bone before rupture of the lesion.

16. Ascaris Intestinal Obstruction

Recipe: Fresh ginger 30 g, and honey 90 g.

Prescription: The ginger juice is mixed with honey for one oral administration. If it is not finished, the remnant may be drunk two hours later.

17. Appendicitis

Recipe 1: An adequate amount of fresh ginger, fresh taro, and wheat flour.

Prescription: The clean and peeled ginger and taro are pounded and mixed with flour to prepare a paste for local application about 3 hours a day.

Explanation: This paste can relieve stagnant blood and stop the pain of acute appendicitis.

Recipe 2: Two portions of garlic and one portion of sodium sulfate and *dahuang* (大 黄, Rhubarb).

Prescription: These herbs are pounded together and mixed with some vinegar to prepare a paste for application over the tender area to the extent of 1-2 cm over 2 hours, after wrapping with a bandage.

Explanation: This method is used to treat appendicitis in the early stages. An operation should be performed in time for patients with suppurative or perforated appendicitis.

18. Retention of Urine

Recipe 1: Green onion 250 g and table salt 500 g.

Prescription: The chopped green onion is fried with salt in a pan and the hot mixture is put into a cloth bag for hot ironing applied arround the umbilicus and lower abdomen. The hot ironing is resumed after the bag is changed several times. This treatment may be continued for 2-3 days until the retention of urine is released.

Explanation: This method can adjust the function of the spleen and stomach and improve kidney function in treating retention of urine after tubercular meningitis, a surgical operation, or a difficult childbirth.

Recipe 2: One bulb of garlic, 7 Cape jasmine, and some salt.

Prescription: The herbs are pounded to prepare a paste and applied over the umbilicus after being spread over a piece of gauze.

Explanation: This method can release obstruction of the urethral orifice to treat retention of urine.

Recipe 3: Three cloves of garlic and 5 mole crickets.

Prescription: The mole crickets and garlic are pounded to prepare a paste for a one-hour application into the umbilicus.

Explanation: This method can release obstruction of the urethral orifice to treat retention of urine and edema.

19. Difficult Urination

Recipe: One clove of new garlic.

Prescription: The garlic is cut into slices and the juice squeezed from the slice is dropped into the meatus of the urethra to produce a stimulating and agitating sensation. The urine may be discharged 10-20 minutes later. If this failed, the treatment may be repeated once more.

Explanation: This method can release obstruction of the urethral orifice to treat postoperative difficult urination.

20. Scrotal Swelling and Pain

Recipe: An adequate amount of green onion stalks and *ruxiang* (乳 香, Frankincense).

Prescription: These herbs are pounded together for application over the scrotum.

Explanation: A decoction of *shechuangzi* (蛇 床 子, Cnidiwn Fruit) 50 g, *kushen* (苦 参, Sophora Root) 50 g, and *wubeizi* (五 倍 子, Chinese Gall) 50 g is used to wash the itching scrotum.

21. Hernia

Recipe 1: Skin of garlic 20 g.

Prescription: A decoction of garlic skin is drunk several times a day.

Explanation: Twenty grams of inner garlic skin can be obtained from 1 kg of garlic, and the decoction can be used to treat hernia in babies.

Recipe 2: An adequate amount of green onion and *zisu* (紫 苏, Perilla Leaf) and a lime bag.

Prescription: The green onion and *zisu* are boiled in water and the warm decoction is used for a sitz bath of 15-20 minutes. The lime bag is put over the affected area during sleep at night.

Explanation: This method may produce a certain effect for treating hernia with distension and pain.

Recipe 3: Fresh ginger 15 g, *danggui* (当 归, Chinese Angelica) 15 g, and mutton 100 g.

Prescription: The ingredients are boiled in water and the well-done meat and soup are taken once a day.

Explanation: This recipe can promote the formation and circulation of blood, release stagnation of qi, control pain, and warm the lower abdomen in treating hernia of the cold type.

Recipe 4: Two bulbs of red-skin garlic, orange seeds 50 g, 2 kumquats, and sugar 50 g.

Prescription: The peeled garlic is boiled with the other ingredients in two bowls of water until one bowl of decoction is obtained for one oral administration.

Explanation: This recipe can resolve swelling and stop pain in treating hernia with severe pain.

Recipe 5: An adequate amount of fresh ginger. Prescription: Ginger is pounded and squeezed to produce juice and the scrotum is immersed in ginger juice for a while.

Explanation: The method can expel cold pathogen from the muscles to treat hernia.

Recipe 6: Outer scales of green onion 90 g.

Prescription: The outer scales of the green onions are boiled in water for one oral administration. This decoction should be taken 7 times.

Explanation: This treatment can expel wind pathogen, induce sweating, relieve toxicity, and resolve swelling in treating hernia.

Recipe 7: Fresh ginger 120 g, 10 pieces of green onion and one bulb of garlic.

Prescription: The ingredients are pounded to prepare a paste for application to the lesion. Hot fried bran is placed into a cloth bag and applied over the paste as a hot compress.

Explanation: This method is used to treat hernia in the early stages.

22. Orchitis

Recipe: An adequate amount of ripe ginger.

Prescription: Eight to ten clean slices of ginger are put on the scrotum which is then wrapped and supported by gauze and bandages for one day.

Explanation: This method can relieve toxicity and inflammation in treating acute orchitis.

23. Swelling of Penis

Recipe: Sticky fluid collected from the tubular leaves of green onion.

Prescription: The fresh leaves of green onion are longitudinally cut open and applied over the penis with the inner mucoid surface in contact with the penis skin for 2 hours after wrapping with a bandage. The therapeutic effect may be detected 4 hours later.

Explanation: This method can moisten dryness and relieve swollen penis.

24. Hemorrhoids

Recipe 1: Roots of green onion 120 g and mirabilite 30 g.

Prescription: A decoction of these ingredients is used to wash the affected area 2-3 times a day for 3 weeks.

Explanation: Hemorrhoids are the soft dilated venous plexuses beneath the mucosa of distal rectum and under the skin of the anal canal. They can be divided into internal, external, and mixed types. This method is used to treat external and mixed hemorrhoids.

Recipe 2: An adequate amount of garlic.

Prescription: The roasted garlic is pounded and wrapped in a piece of gauze for application as a local hot compress.

Explanation: This is a folk treatment used in Japan for hemorrhoids.

Recipe 3: Three pieces of green onion, pepper 2 g, *caoguo* (草 果, Tsaoko) powder 1 g, and one large fresh crucian carp.

Prescription: The fish is washed and cut into slices and the pepper is ground into powder. The fish is boiled with the herbs and condiments as a dish taken before meals.

Explanation: This fish dish is used for chronic hemorrhoids with bleeding.

Recipe 4: An adequate amount of garlic.

Prescription: The garlic paste or juice is diluted with 3-5 times the volume of water for application with cotton balls over the affected area.

Explanation: This method can resolve swelling, relieve stagnant blood, and stop bleeding.

Recipe 5: An adequate amount of onion and honey.

Prescription: The onion and honey are pounded to prepare a paste for application to the hemorrhoids to resolve swelling and stop pain.

Explanation: This is a good method for treating swollen and painful hemorrhoids.

25. Pain and Swelling of Limbs

Recipe: Green onion 100 g, 4 pig's feet and some salt.

Prescription: The cleaned pig's feet are stewed with green onion and salt until the meat is softened for oral administration with soup, twice a day.

Explanation: This meat dish can clear heat and resolve swelling to treat pain, edema, and ulcers of the limbs due to blood deficiency.

Chapter 4
GYNECOLOGICAL DISEASES

1. Dysmenorrhea

Recipe 1: Fresh ginger cut into bits 120 g; 49 green onion stalks, washed and pounded, and salt 500 g.

Prescription: These ingredients are fried in a pot and wrapped in a towel as a hot compress applied over the painful area.

Explanation: Periodic pain of the lower abdomen and waist, sometimes intractable and recurrent, before, during or after the menstrual period, is called dysmenorrhea.

Recipe 2: Fresh ginger 15 g, and brown sugar 15 g.

Prescription: A hot water decoction of these ingredients is orally administered, twice a day.

Explanation: This decoction is very effective in treating dysmenorrhea due to cold stagnation and dampness, and deficiency of qi and blood.

Recipe 3: Fresh ginger 9 g, *muxiang* (木 香 , Costus Root) 6 g, and fennel 15 g.

Prescription: A decoction of these herbs is orally administered.

Explanation: This recipe is mainly used to treat dysmenorrhea with abdominal pain due to stagnation of cold and dampness.

Recipe 4: One piece of fresh ginger, 3-5 green onion stalks with roots, brown sugar 150 g, and one spoonful of pepper powder.

Prescription: The crushed ginger, green onion, and brown sugar are boiled in 2 bowls of water for 5-8 minutes and the hot decoction is taken after the pepper powder is added. It may be taken once more a few hours later if the abdominal pain is not relieved, and it may be taken three times a day until the pain stops.

Explanation: This recipe can be used to treat dysmenorrhea and stasis of blood after child birth.

Recipe 5: Fresh ginger 10-15 g, *aiye* (艾 叶, Leaf of Mugwort) 10-15 g, and an adequate amount of brown sugar.

Prescription: A hot decoction of the ingredients is orally administered, 2 times a day.

Explanation: This recipe is used to treat dysmenorrhea with abdominal pain caused by cold stagnation and damp and relievable by heat. The menstrual discharge is dark, scanty, and mixed with blood clots.

2. Amenorrhea

Recipe 1: Fresh ginger 25 g, brown sugar 100 g, and red dates 100 g.

Prescription: A tea is made with the ingredients for constant drinking until menstruation recurs.

Explanation: This tea can nourish the blood, promote blood circulation, expel cold pathogen, and adjust meridians in treating amenorrhea.

Recipe 2: Fresh ginger 25 g, *danggui* (当 归, Chinese Angelica) 25 g, and lean pork meat 200 g.

Prescription: The meat is well cooked with ginger and *danggui* for oral administration with the soup, once a day.

Explanation: This preparation can nourish spleen qi and stomach and warm the abdominal organs in treating amenorrhea with abdominal pain due to blood exhaustion, blood deficiency after child birth, and consumptive diseases in women.

Recipe 3: Fresh ginger 9 g, parched *aiye* (艾 叶, Leaf of

Mugwort) 9 g, and *rougui* (肉 桂, Chinese Cinnamon Bark) 6 g.

Prescription: A water decoction of these herbs is orally administered.

Explanation: Amenorrhea may appear in pre-adolescent young girls or in women whose regular menstruation has stopped for over 3 months.

3. Oligomenorrhea

Recipe: Garlic of good quality 700 g and liquor 1.8 liters over 40 degrees centigrade.

Prescription: The clean peeled garlic is dried in shadow and then pounded and mixed with liquor in a bottle filled 90 percent. After storage in the cellar for 3 months to 3 years, the garlic extract is filtered and diluted with twice the amount of water for oral administration of one cup, twice a day, after mixing with crystal sugar or honey. Crystal sugar 75 g or one cup of honey is dissolved in 1.8 liters of garlic extract. Vital energy may be much improved after administration of this preparation for one week, any menstruation may return to normal after administration for 1-3 months.

Explanation: This alcohol extract of garlic can enhance hemopoiesis and improve ovary function to treat oligomenorrhea and infertility due to anemia in women.

4. Profuse Uterine Bleeding

Recipe 1: Three pieces of green onion, ginger 50 g, two unfertilized chicken eggs, and an adequate amount of sesame oil.

Prescription: The green onion, ginger, and eggs are pounded and fried in sesame oil for oral administration with hot wine after the ginger and green onion are removed.

Explanation: This recipe is used to treat profuse uterine bleeding over a long time due to a deficiency of qi and blood.

Recipe 2: Ginger charcoal 30 g and *fulonggan* (伏 龙 肝, Calcined Yellow Earth) 60 g.

Prescription: These herbs are boiled in 2 bowls of water to prepare one-bowl decoction, and the supernatant liquid is taken orally.

Explanation: The ginger charcoal is prepared by baking the ginger in an earth pot until the ginger skin turns dark brown. This recipe is used to treat profuse uterine bleeding or persistent dribbling of uterine blood.

5. Menstrual Stomachache

Recipe: Ginger 25 g, 3 duck eggs with light blue shells and yellow wine 250 g.

Prescription: The eggs and ginger are boiled in yellow wine for oral administration.

Explanation: This preparation can warm internal organs, expel cold pathogen, adjust meridians, and stop pain in the treatment of poor appetite and pain in the stomach, lower abdomen, and waist during the menstrual period.

6. Menstrual Vomiting

Recipe: Dried ginger 2.5 g, cloves 2.5 g, and *baizhu* (白 术, Largehead Atractylodis) 50 g.

Prescription: The herbs are pounded to make a powder preparation and divided into 10 portions for oral administration of one portion with thin rice gruel in the morning for 10 days, and even longer until the suffering is relieved.

Explanation: This is a safe recipe without side effects. It is also useful for treating abdominal pain and vomiting due to other causes.

7. Leukorrheal Disorders

Recipe 1: Dried ginger 3 g and limonite 30 g.

Prescription: These herbs are ground to make a powder

preparation for oral administration of 6 g with yellow wine, twice a day.

Explanation: This recipe is used to treat various leukorrheal disorders.

Recipe 2: Dried ginger 10 g, fennel 20 g, and an adequate amount of brown sugar.

Prescription: A decoction of these herbs is prepared for oral administration.

Explanation: This recipe is used to treat grave leukorrhea.

Recipe 3: Dried ginger 15 g, and *baishao* (白 芍, White Peony Root) 30 g.

Prescription: The herbs are ground and fried to prepare a light yellow powder for oral administration of 6 g before meals, twice a day with thin rice gruel, for half a month.

Explanation: This recipe is used to treat red and white leukorrhea and abdominal pain around the umbilicus.

8. Pregnancy Vomiting

Recipe 1: One spoonful of fresh ginger juice and one cup of sugarcane juice.

Prescription: A hot mixture of these two juices is taken orally.

Explanation: This mixed juice can improve stomach function, transport qi downward, and control vomiting in treating pregnancy vomiting and difficult swallowing.

Recipe 2: Fresh ginger 200 g, Chinese chives 200 g, and sugar.

Prescription: The chives and ginger are cut into bits and pounded to make juice for oral administration after mixing with sugar.

Explanation: This juice can warm the spleen and stomach, stop vomiting, promote circulation of qi, and adjust spleen and stomach functions in treating nausea, vomiting, and poor appetite after pregnancy.

Recipe 3: Fresh ginger 15 g, radish seeds 15 g, and shaddock skin 15 g.

Prescription: The ingredients are boiled in one bowl of water to prepare half a bowl of decoction for oral administration.

Explanation: This recipe can warm the spleen and stomach and stop vomiting during pregnancy.

Recipe 4: Fresh ginger 5 g, and *Fulonggan* (伏 龙 肝 , Calcined Yellow Earth) 30 g.

Prescription: A decoction of these ingredients is taken orally.

Explanation: Pernicious vomiting during pregnancy with nausea, dizziness, and anorexia is caused by an impairment of the transporting function of the stomach and an adverse ascent of qi in the Chong (vital) meridian.

Recipe 5: Fresh ginger 12 g, *fuling* (茯 苓 , Poria Coccus) 12 g, and *banxia* (半 夏 , Ternate Pinellia) 6 g.

Prescription: A decoction of these herbs is administered orally.

Explanation: This mixture may stop nausea and vomiting of the early stage pregnant.

Recipe 6: Fresh ginger 30 g and sugar 30 g.

Prescription: A decoction of these ingredients is taken orally.

Explanation: This mixture may produce a good effect to stop pregnancy vomiting if constantly drunk for one entire day.

Recipe 7: Ripe ginger 9 g and shaddock skin 18 g.

Prescription: The ginger slices and shaddock skin are boiled in one cup of water to obtain half a cup of decoction and the cool decoction is administered orally after the dregs are removed.

Explanation: The ginger can control vomiting and the shaddock skin can depress the adverse ascent of qi in treating pregnancy vomiting. This decoction should be taken in moderation because of its irritant nature.

9. Pregnancy Diarrhea

Recipe: Equal amounts of dried ginger and *houpo* (厚 朴 ,

Magnolia Bark).

Prescription: After removing the skin, the *houpo* is pounded with dried ginger to make a powder preparation. The fried dry powder is boiled with wheat flour to prepare pills the size of Chinese parasol tree seeds, for oral administration of 50 pills with thin rice gruel before meals.

Explanation: This preparation is used to treat pregnancy diarrhea caused by cold pathogen.

10. Pregnancy Restlessness

Recipe: One handful of green onion stalks and *dandouchi* (淡豆豉, Medicated Soybean) 30 g.

Prescription: These herbs are boiled in 500 ml of water to obtain a decoction of 350 ml for three oral administrations after warming.

Explanation: This recipe is used to treat anxiety and hot sensations in pregnant women.

11. Habitual Abortion

Recipe: One green onion stalk and an adequate amount of *fulonggan* (伏龙肝, Calcined Yellow Earth) and *aiye* (艾叶, Leaf of Mugwort).

Prescription: A decoction of these ingredients is orally administered.

Explanation: This recipe is used to treat habitual abortion.

12. Vaginal Bleeding During Pregnancy

Recipe 1: Green onion stalks 100 g, and *chuanxiong* (川芎, Rhizome) 10 g.

Prescription: The oral administration of a concentrated decoction of green onion stalks may stop vaginal bleeding in pregnant women. If bleeding could not stop *chuanxiong* and rice 50 g may be added to cook a rice soup for oral administration.

Explanation: Vaginal bleeding during pregnancy could be a

symptom of impending abortion and should be treated seriously.

Recipe 2: An adequate amount of dried ginger and *dihuang* (地 黄 , Rehmannia Root).

Prescription: These herbs are ground to a powder preparation for oral administration of 6 g with wine.

Explanation: This recipe is used to treat vaginal bleeding in pregnant women to prevent abortion.

13. Threatened Abortion

Recipe 1: An adequate amount of green onion, ginger, and one perch.

Prescription: After removing the internal organs and washing clean, the fish is boiled with green onion and ginger for about one hour. The fish meat and soup is taken, 3 times a day.

Explanation: Frequent intake of perch can prevent abortion and promote urination to treat threatened abortion and pregnancy edema.

Recipe 2: Green onion stalks 30 g, *dandouchi* (淡 豆 豉 , Medicated Soybean) 30 g, and fried donkey skin gel 60 g.

Prescription: The green onion and *douchi* are boiled in 3,000 ml of water until 1,000 ml of decoction is obtained. The donkey skin gel is added to the boiled decoction after the dregs are removed for oral administration, 3-4 times a day.

Explanation: This recipe is used to treat threatened abortion.

14. Retention of Lochia

Recipe: Juice of fresh ginger 40 ml, juice of *dihuang* (地 黄 , Rehmannia Root) 60 ml, and rice 60 g.

Prescription: The ginger juice and *dihuang* are taken orally with rice soup before sleep.

Explanation: This mixture can promote the discharge of lochia (blood, mucus, and dead uterine mucosa from the vagina).

15. Retention of Placenta

Recipe: Green onion stalks 120-250 g.

Prescription: A hot concentrated decoction of green onion is used to wash the perineum.

Explanation: Retention of placenta is the delayed delivery of the placenta after childbirth.

16. Postpartum Vomiting

Recipe: Fresh ginger 1.8 g and *baizhu* (白 术 , Largehead Atractylodis) 1.5 g.

Prescription: These herbs are cut into fine bits and boiled in 2,000 ml of water after mixing with wine to prepare a decoction of 1,000 ml for oral administration, 3 times.

Explanation: This recipe is used to treat vomiting and poor appetite after childbirth.

17. Postpartum Abdominal Pain

Recipe 1: Fresh ginger 30 g, *danggui* (当 归 , Chinese Angelicae) 60 g, and fatty mutton 120 g.

Prescription: The decoction of ginger and *danggui* is used to cook mutton for oral administration before breakfast in an amount according to the patient's appetite.

Explanation: If the abdominal pain of childbirth lasts for an abnormal length of time after delivery, this is known as postpartum abdominal pain.

Recipe 2: Powder of dried ginger 1.5 g and brown sugar 25 g.

Prescription: The ingredients are dissolved in hot boiled water as a tea for repeated drinking.

Explanation: This recipe can warm the spleen and stomach, expel cold pathogen, promote blood circulation, and relieve stagnant blood in treating postpartum abdominal pain.

Recipe 3: Stored ginger 250 g and prepared *dihuang* (地 黄 , Rehmannia Root) 500 g.

Prescription: These herbs are ground into powder for oral administration of 10 g with warm wine.

Explanation: The ginger can warm meridians and expel cold pathogen, and the prepared *dihuang* can nourish yin and blood to treat postpartum abdominal pain due to blood loss and blood.

18. Postpartum Edema

Recipe: Juice of fresh ginger 90 g, wheat flour 90 g, and 7 pieces of *banxia* (半 夏 , Ternate Pinellia).

Prescription: The *banxia* is wrapped with a paste made of flour and ginger juice and roasted over fire until it is charred to prepare powder for oral administration after mixing with 250 ml of water. This preparation can induce the discharge of urine.

Explanation: This recipe is used to treat postpartum edema and asthma.

19. Postpartum Fainting

Recipe 1: Four slices of fresh ginger, wheat 20 g, and 7 red dates.

Prescription: A decoction of these herbs is taken orally.

Explanation: Some women after childbirth are unable to sit up and may suddenly develop dizziness, vertigo, nausea, and even delirium and unconsciousness.

Recipe 2: Three green onion stalks and glutinous rice 60 g.

Prescription: These ingredients are boiled to cook a rice soup for oral administration every day.

Explanation: This recipe may also be used to treat threatened abortion in the first few months of pregnancy.

20. Postpartum Weakness

Recipe 1: Fresh ginger juice 100 g, lard 100 g, and yellow wine 50 ml.

Prescription: These ingredients are boiled and stored in bottles for use after cooling. One spoonful of the oily paste is melted in boiled water for oral administration, twice a day.

Explanation: This recipe can nourish yin, clear heat, and relieve weakness in treating postpartum weakness with spontaneous sweating and alternate attacks of chills and fever.

Recipe 2: Fresh ginger 300 g and 2 pig's feet.

Prescription: The peeled ginger and pig's feet are cut into lumps and cooked in 600 ml of sweet vinegar for oral administration over several days.

Explanation: As a good tonic for women after childbirth, this brew can strengthen the spleen and stomach, nourish qi and blood, promote the discharge of milk, and remove stagnant blood.

Recipe 3: Fresh ginger 30 g, flowering quince fruit 500 g, and vinegar 500 ml.

Prescription: The ingredients are stewed in a mud pot and stored for several oral administration.

Explanation: This is a folk remedy for women after childbirth to restore their spirit and energy, reinforce contraction of the uterus, promote discharge of lochia, and release stagnant blood. It is also useful to increase the discharge of milk.

21. Oligogalactia

Recipe: An adequate amount of green onion stalks and *wangbuliuxing* (王 不 留 行, Cow Soupwort Seed) 30 g.

Prescription: A decoction of these herbs is taken orally.

Explanation: This recipe is used to treat oligogalactia due to general weakness, reduced formation of qi and blood, or blockage of milk discharge due to stagnation of liver qi.

22. Breast Cancer

Recipe: Five large slices of fresh ginger, 7 green onion stalks, *fangfeng* (防 风, Saposhnikovia Root) 3 g, and *beimu* (贝 母, Bulb of Fritillary) 9 g.

Prescription: These herbs are boiled in 500 ml of water to

obtain 350 ml of decoction, and boiled again in water to obtain a second portion of decoction. The two portions are mixed together for two oral administrations after the decoction is warmed to induce sweating. The pounded dregs are applied over the breast tumor and covered with paper.

23. Hysteria

Recipe: Dried ginger 3 g, white pepper 3 g, and one chicken egg.

Prescription: A hole is made in the egg shell and the powder of ginger and pepper is put into the shell. The egg is then stewed after the hole is sealed. The stewed egg is orally administered with yellow wine.

Explanation: Women with hysteria may have symptoms of mental depression, restlessness, unreasonable laughing and crying, and repeated yawning.

24. Vulvar Itching

Recipe 1: Five stalks of green onion and niter 6 g.

Prescription: A decoction of these ingredients is used to wash the perineal region.

Explanation: Intractable itching and pain of the vulva and vagina are common symptoms in women with restlessness and the disturbance of leukorrhea. This method may also be used to treat vulvar pain.

Recipe 2: Two bulbs of garlic.

Prescription: A decoction of garlic paste is used to wash the perineal region or for a sitz bath, 2-3 times a day.

Explanation: The garlic can kill bacteria, control inflammation, and stop itching.

25. Infertility

Recipe 1: Green onion stalks 60 g, ripe ginger 20 g, *aiye* (艾 叶, Leaf of Mugwort) 60 g, and peeled dried fowel gourd

60 g.

Prescription: These herbs are fried and wrapped in gauze for a hot compress applied to the lower abdomen, once a day.

Explanation: This method is used to treat infertility due to blood, kidney, and spleen deficiency.

Recipe 2: Fresh ginger 500 g and brown sugar 500 g.

Prescription: In the hottest part of summer, the ginger paste and sugar are steamed for one hour and sundried for three days. Then the preparation is repeatedly steamed and sundried a total of nine times. One spoonful of this preparation is orally administered, 3 times a day, from the first day of menstruation for one month. During the treatment, sexual intercourse is prohibited.

Explanation: This preparation can expel wind and cold pathogen, warm the uterus, and promote blood circulation in treating infertility due to cold in the uterus.

Chapter 5
PEDIATRIC DISEASES

1. Common Cold in Newborn Babies

Recipe 1: An adequate amount of fresh ginger and one large *tiannanxing* (天 南 星, Jack-in-the-Pulpit).

Prescription: A powder of *tiannanxing* is mixed with ginger juice to prepare a paste for application over the fontanel.

Explanation: The local application of this paste should only last a short time.

Recipe 2: An adequate amount of green onion, *caowu* (草 乌, Wild Aconite Root) and *zaojiao* (皂 草, Chinese Honey Locust).

Prescription: A powder of *caowu* and *zaojiao* is mixed with green onion juice to prepare a paste for application over the fontanel.

Explanation: This paste is used to treat the common colds in newborn infants. It should not be applied in large amounts or for a long time.

2. Common Cold in Children

Recipe 1: Fresh ginger 15-30 g, and brown sugar 20 g.

Prescription: The clean ginger slices are pounded and boiled in water with brown sugar for oral administration of 50-100 ml while still hot.

Explanation: This decoction can expel wind and cold pathogen in treating common clods in children caused by an attack of wind and cold pathogen.

116

Recipe 2: An adequate amount of green onion stalks.

Prescription: After washing clean and cutting into small bits, the green onion is soaked in boiled water for inhalation of the hot steam. The child is asked to take deep breaths.

Explanation: This method can open orifices of the sense organs and remove pathogens from the muscles in treating the common cold in children.

Recipe 3: An adequate amount of green onion stalks.

Prescription: The clean green onion is pounded and the juice is applied over the upper lip.

Explanation: This method can open orifices of the sense organs and expel pathogen from the body's surface in treating the common cold in infants with nasal obstruction and difficulty sucking milk.

3. Bronchitis in Children

Recipe 1: Fresh ginger 3 g, tea leaves 3 g, and brown sugar 9 g.

Prescription: A decoction of these herbs is orally administered, 3 times a day.

Explanation: This recipe is used to treat bronchitis with fever, cough, and asthma.

Recipe 2: Fresh ginger 3 g, *shegan* (射 干 , Blackberry Lily) 3 g, and *jingjie* (荆 芥 , Schizonepeta) 3 g.

Prescription: A decoction of these herbs is orally administered.

Explanation: This recipe can warm the spleen and stomach, expel cold pathogen, and control cough and asthma in treating bronchitis in children.

Recipe 3: Fresh ginger 3 slices, honey 20 ml, and frost of dry persimmon 6 g.

Prescription: The ingredients are mixed and steamed for over 20 minutes for one oral administration, 1-2 times a day.

Explanation: This recipe can moisten the lungs, stop cough,

warm the spleen and stomach, expel cold pathogen, and relieve exterior syndrome.

4. Asthma in Children

Recipe: Garlic 500 g, 4 egg yolks, and calcium powder 20 g.

Prescription: The garlic is cut into fine bits and boiled in a pan with a small amount of water for 2 hours to prepare a paste which is then mixed with the egg yolks. After boiling on a low fire, the garlic paste and egg yolks are mixed with calcium powder to prepare pills for oral administration, one pill a day.

Explanation: The garlic can improve appetite, promote metabolism and circulation of qi and blood, and control allergies. At the same time, it can also affect bacteria in the intestines to produce thiamine.

5. Pneumonia in Children

Recipe: Garlic 30 g.

Prescription: Garlic paste is soaked in boiled water for half an hour and taken orally after mixing with cane sugar when it is still warm and after the dregs are removed, 4 times a day for 7 days.

Explanation: This method can relieve all symptoms of pneumonia in children.

6. Whooping Cough

Recipe 1: Garlic 60 g, and an adequate amount of sugar.

Prescription: The peeled garlic is cut into small bits and soaked in cold boiled water for 10 hours. The extract is administered orally with some sugar once every 2 hours in a dosage of 15 ml for patients above 5 years old, and one half of this dosage for children below 5 years of age.

Explanation: This method can control cough and promote the discharge of sputum for treating whooping cough in children. During an epidemic of whooping cough, the garlic extract can also be used to prevent infections from this disease.

Recipe 2: An adequate amount of green onion leaves, bean curd, and crystal sugar.

Prescription: The crystal sugar is put into the tubular green onion leaves, which are then put into the bean curd and steamed until the sugar is melted. The steamed green onion with sugar juice is orally administered twice a day, 3 leaves for one oral administration in babies below 2 years old, and 5-7 leaves in children above 2 years of age. *Beimu* (贝 母, Fritillary) 3-6 g may be added to the preparation in patients with spastic cough.

Explanation: This preparation can control cough and asthma in treating whooping cough.

Recipe 3: One bulb of garlic with purple skin and one dried orange.

Prescription: These ingredients are boiled in one bowl of water for oral administration, 2-3 times a day, after the dregs are removed and some honey is added.

Explanation: This is a useful method for treating whooping cough in children. In addition, before going to bed the garlic paste is spread over a piece of gauze in a thickness of one mm and applied over the soles of the feet which are protected by applying a layer of vaseline. The garlic paste over the soles is covered with a piece of plastic membrane and kept in position by putting on socks; it is removed the next morning. If no pain is caused by the garlic paste, this treatment may be continued for 3-5 days, or applied once every 2 days. This treatment can also be used to treat night cough due to other diseases.

Recipe 4: Fresh ginger 40 g, pig lung 20 g, and tea leaves 25 g.

Prescription: The ginger and pig lung are pounded and then boiled in water with tea leaves to prepare a decoction for oral administration.

Explanation: This recipe can nourish yin and moisten lungs to treat late-stage whooping cough in children.

7. Chronic Cough in Children

Recipe: Garlic 20 g, and honey 15 g.

Prescription: The garlic paste is soaked in a cup of water and boiled for over one hour for oral administration after mixing with honey.

Explanation: This recipe can clear heat, moisten the lungs, kill bacteria, and control inflammation in treating children with uncontrollable cough and insomnia.

8. Diarrhea in Children

Recipe 1: One bulb of garlic.

Prescription: The charred garlic with its therapeutic effect preserved is soaked in boiled water. The garlic extract is orally administered several times a day.

Explanation: This method is particularly useful for treating chronic diarrhea in children.

Recipe 2: Fresh ginger fried with salt 6 g, red dates 6 g, and brown sugar 6 g.

Prescription: The ginger and dates are boiled in water for 50 minutes and then continuously boiled for a short time after brown sugar is added. The decoction is orally administered in the morning and at night.

Explanation: This recipe is used to treat diarrhea in children.

Recipe 3: Green onion stalks 12 g, fresh ginger 6 g, aiye (艾 叶 , Leaf of Mugwort) 20 g, and cactus root 30 g.

Prescription: These herbs are pounded and mixed with egg white to prepare a paste for application over the umbilical region.

Explanation: This method is used to treat diarrhea in children caused by external pathogen.

Recipe 4: An adequate amount of ginger.

Prescription: The charred ginger is ground to produce a powder preparation for oral administration with thin rice gruel.

Explanation: This preparation is used to treat diarrhea with bloody stool caused by enteritis in children.

9. Indigestion in Children

Recipe 1: Fresh ginger 1 g, *banxia* (半 夏, Ternate Pinellia) 6 g, and *fuling* (茯 苓, Poria) 4.5 g.

Prescription: A decoction of these ingredients is drunk 3 times.

Explanation: This recipe is used to treat indigestion in babies with bluish stool and regurgitation of milk.

Recipe 2: An adequate amount of green onion stalks and white turnip.

Prescription: These two vegetables are washed clean, cut into small bits, and pounded to produce a juice for oral administration.

Explanation: This juice can promote digestion, release stagnation of food, and transport gas downward for treating indigestion and food stagnation in children.

10. Constipation in Children

Recipe: Three green onion stalks and an adequate amount of honey.

Prescription: The paste of green onion is mixed with honey for application over the umbilicus. The thick end of the green onion is inserted into the anus after dipping in honey to induce bowel movement.

Explanation: This methods can produce a good effect in treating constipation in children.

11. Abdominal Pain in Children

Recipe: Fresh ginger 20 g, green onion stalks 20 g and *dandouchi* (淡 豆 豉, Medicated Soybean) 20 g.

Prescription: These herbs are cut into small bits and fried with half a bowel of salt for application as a hot compress over the umbilical region with the hot material wrapped in a towel.

Explanation: This method is used in treating crying babies with bodies bent by abdominal pain.

12. Vomiting in Children

Recipe 1: An adequate amount of fresh ginger, one red date, and *dingxiang* (丁 香, cloves) 1 g.

Prescription: A decoction of these herbs is orally administered.

Explanation: This recipe is particularly useful for treating milk regurgitation

Recipe 2: An adequate amount of ginger juice and powder of *geqiao* (蛤 壳, Clam Shell) 12 g.

Prescription: A powder of *geqiao* is mixed with ginger juice to make a paste for application over the Yongquan (KI 1) acupoint.

Explanation: This method is used to treat regurgitation of milk. The Yongquan acupoints are at the center of the soles (at the junction of anterior one third and posterior two thirds of sole).

Recipe 3: Fresh ginger 3 g, one red date, and some brown sugar.

Prescription: A decoction of the ingredients is orally administered.

Explanation: This recipe is used to treat regurgitation of milk or vomiting in young children due to improper feeding, stagnation of food, and weakness and cold of the spleen and stomach.

Recipe 4: Two green onion stalks and an adequate amount of human milk.

Prescription: The green onion stalks are stewed with human milk for oral administration.

Explanation: This preparation can warm and adjust the spleen and stomach to treat regurgitation of milk due to weakness and cold in the spleen and stomach.

Recipe 5: One lump of fresh ginger and 1 grain of *dingxiang* (丁 香 , cloves).

Prescription: A small hole is made in the ginger and the *dingxiang* is placed into the small hole. Then the ginger is boiled in water after the hole is sealed and the decoction is administered orally.

Explanation: This method can warm and adjust the spleen and stomach, expel cold pathogen, and dispel weakness in treating regurgitation of milk in babies caused by an attack of wind and cold pathogen.

13. Food Stagnation in Children

Recipe 1: Green onion stalks 6 g and human milk 30 g.

Prescription: A water decoction of these ingredients is orally administered.

Explanation: This method is used to treat food stagnation and poor appetite due to indigestion.

Recipe 2: Dried ginger 3 g, *baizhi* (白 芷 , Chinese Angelicae) 3 g, and *wubeizi* (五 倍 子 , Chinese Gall, baked to a yellow color) 9 g.

Prescription: The herbs are ground to prepare powder for oral administration of 3 g, 2 times a day for babies one year old, and larger doses for older children.

Explanation: This powder can also be applied to the umbilicus and covered with adhesive plaster to treat indigestion in children.

Recipe 3: An adequate amount of fresh ginger and *zisu* (紫 苏 , Perilla Leaf).

Prescription: These herbs are pounded and fried hot for repeated application as a hot compress over the chest and abdomen.

Explanation: This method is used to treat stagnation of clod and indigestible food in children.

14. Infantile Malnutrition

Recipe 1: One spoonful of ginger juice, 2 grains of *dingxiang* (丁 香 , cloves), and cow milk 250 ml.

Prescription: The ingredients are stewed in a pot for oral administration after the *dingxiang* is removed and some sugar is added.

Explanation: This recipe can dispel weakness, depress adverse ascending qi, control vomiting, and stop pain in treating emaciated children who vomit right after eating.

Recipe 2: Fresh ginger 6 g, green onion stalks 1 g, *ganjicao* (疳积草) 60 g, and one egg white.

Prescription: The pounded herbs are mixed with egg white for application over the soles of the feet.

Explanation: This method is used to treat indigestive malnutrition due to stagnation of qi and food in the stomach and intestines.

Recipe 3: Two cloves of garlic and an adequate amount of *cheqianzi* (车 前 子 , Plantain Seed, fried and ground).

Prescription: These ingredients are pounded to prepare a paste for application into the umbilicus for about 4 hours.

Explanation: This method is used to treat malnutrition in children with abdominal distension.

15. Parasitic Diseases in Children

Recipe 1: One handful of green onion stalks and 1-2 spoonfuls of sesame or rape seed oil.

Prescription: The green onion is washed and cut into bits to obtain juice by squeezing. After mixing with oil, the preparation is orally administered before meals, twice a day for 3 successive days.

Explanation: This recipe can expel parasites and stop pain in treating abdominal pain caused by ascaris.

Recipe 2: An adequate amount of garlic and vaseline.

Prescription: The mixture of garlic paste and vaseline is

applied around the the anus before going to bed and washed away the next morning.

Explanation: This method is used to treat pinworm with itching around the anus.

Recipe 3: An adequate amount of garlic.

Prescription: The garlic juice is orally administered for several days to expel parasites.

Explanation: This method is used to treat ascariasis. Some brown granulated sugar may be added to modify the peppery taste of garlic.

Recipe 4: An adequate amount of garlic and soybean sauce.

Prescription: These ingredients are stewed for oral administration of 2-3 cloves of garlic before meals, 3 times a day.

Explanation: This method is used to treat pinworm.

Recipe 5: Fresh ginger 60 g, and honey 60 ml.

Prescription: The ginger juice and honey are mixed for oral administration of a daily dosage of 30-40 ml in children 1-4 years old; 50 ml in children 5-6 years old; and 50-60 ml in children 7-13 years old. The total of 120 ml of mixed juice is taken over 2-3 times.

Explanation: This recipe can warm and adjust the spleen and stomach and control vomiting and pain in treating intestinal obstruction caused by ascaris. In general, the abdominal mass may disappear after administration of this juice, and then the antiscolic drug may be administered. When treated with this juice, the patient must be carefully watched and should immediately seek surgery if the intestinal gurgling sound disappears.

Recipe 6: Green onion 50 g.

Prescription: The clean green onion is boiled in 100 ml of water on a low flame until very soft. The liquid is then stored in a bottle for use after filtering with gauze. The liquid is used for enemas before going to bed, 10 ml of liquid for children 4-5 years old, and 15 ml for children 6 years old and over.

Explanation: This method is used to treat pinworm in young

children. Garlic may be used instead, but the garlic should be boiled in 200 ml of water.

Recipe 7: Garlic 9 g, Chinese torreya seed 9 g, and almond 4.5 g.

Prescription: The torreya seed and almond are ground to make fine powder and mixed with garlic paste to prepare pills for two oral administrations with boiled water.

Explanation: This pill is used to treat tapeworm due to infected pork or beef with encysted cercaria.

16. Foul Smell from Mouth in Children

Recipe: Fresh ginger juice 10 ml and cow milk 20 ml.

Prescription: These liquids are boiled for a while in a silver container on a low flame for oral administration.

Explanation: The dosage for one-year-old babies is 10 ml. This can be increased for older children.

17. Dribbling of Saliva in Children

Recipe: Fresh ginger 3 g, and *gancao* (甘 草 , Licorice) 6 g.

Prescription: A decoction of these herbs is orally administered.

Explanation: This is a symptom in young children below 3 years old, with profuse excretion of saliva and flushing and chafed chin. But it is a normal phenomenon in teething children.

18. Aphtha in Children

Recipe: Dried ginger 1.5 g and *huanglian* (黄 连 , Goldthread)) 1.5 g.

Prescription: A powder of these herbs is applied over the affected area, 2-3 times a day.

Explanation: This is a common disease of the mouth cavity in children, characterized by small pale yellow or white ulcers of varied size on the buccal mucosa, tongue, and gum.

19. Incontinence of Urine in Children

Recipe: Seven to eight green onion stalks and sulfur 50 g.

Prescription: These two ingredients are pounded to prepare a juice for application over the umbilicus before going to bed for three successive nights.

Explanation: This method can nourish yang and heat in treating incontinence of urine.

20. Retention of Urine in Children

Recipe 1: An adequate amount of garlic.

Prescription: The garlic paste is spread over paper and applied over the lower abdomen below the umbilicus.

Explanation: The garlic paste should be immediately removed right after the urine is discharged to prevent formation of blisters.

Recipe 2: A green onion stalk of 9-12 cm in length, and an adequate amount of human milk.

Prescription: The paste of green onion is mixed with human milk and put into the child's mouth for sucking to induce discharge of urine.

Explanation: This method is used in treating retention of urine in newborn babies.

21. Epidemic Parotitis

Recipe 1: Fresh ginger juice 50 ml, vinegar 50 ml, and pig bile 3 ml.

Prescription: These ingredients are mixed together and applied over the lesion.

Explanation: Parotitis is an acute epidemic disease of the respiratory system common in children with fever, pain, and swollen parotid gland caused by the virus of epidemic parotitis.

Recipe 2: Equal amounts of garlic and vinegar.

Prescription: The garlic is pounded with vinegar to prepare a paste for application over the lesion, 2-4 times a day until the swelling is resolved. Paste used for application over the affected area should be newly prepared.

Explanation: This method is used to treat epidemic parotitis in the early stages. Drugs for oral administration may be used in combination with this method, if the patient has fever, headache, and other general symptoms.

Recipe 3: Two green onion stalks and raw *dahuang* (大 黄, Rhubarb) 30 g.

Prescription: The green onion is pounded and mixed with *dahuang* powder to prepare a paste for application over the lesion, once a day.

Explanation: This recipe can relieve toxicity, remove stagnation, and clear heat.

Recipe 4: Three green onion stalks.

Prescription: The green onion is cut and pounded to prepare a paste for application over the lesion.

Explanation: This method can relieve stagnation and resolve swelling in treating epidemic parotitis.

Recipe 5: An adequate amount of ginger juice and *dahuang* (大 黄, Rhubarb) powder.

Prescription: A paste of these ingredients is applied over the parotid gland, except at the center of the gland. The swollen gland may gradually resolve in a few days.

Explanation: This method can clear heat and remove stagnation to effectively treat epidemic parotitis.

22. Measles in Children

Recipe: A handful of green onion stalks and a handful of coriander.

Prescription: A decoction of these two ingredients is used to wash and rub the entire body, especially the precordial region, palms, and soles of the feet.

Explanation: This method can promote the healing of the skin rash.

23. Convulsions in Children

Recipe 1: Dried ginger 9 g, *rougui* (肉 桂 , Chinese Cinnamon Bark) 9 g, and *wuzhuyu* (吴 茱 萸 , Evodia Fruit) 9 g.

Prescription: These herbs are ground to make a powder preparation for oral administration of 3 g, two times a day in one-year-old babies, for 5-6 days.

Explanation: Convulsion is a common symptom in children between 1-5 years old. The incidence is higher in younger children, and much reduced after 7 years of age. Convulsions can be divided into acute and chronic types, and this recipe is used to treat chronic convulsions.

Recipe 2: Dried ginger 6 g, *xixin* (细 辛 , Wild Ginger) 3 g, and *zhuyazao* (猪 牙 皂 , Chinese Honey Locust) 9 g.

Prescription: A powder of these herbs is snorted into the nostrils to induce sneezing.

Explanation: This recipe is used to treat acute convulsions.

Recipe 3: A large green onion stalks, fresh ginger 5 g, distiller's grains 50 g, and 7-11 willow tree twigs (about 6-7 cm long).

Prescription: After the core and rough skin of the willow twigs are removed, these ingredients are pounded and fried (not in an iron utensil) and then the hot material is spread over a piece of cotton cloth for application over the fontanel of the sick baby for 20-30 minutes

Explanation: This method is used to treat convulsions in babies due to high fever.

24. Night Crying

Recipe 1: One green onion stalks, 3 grains of pepper, and 3 pieces of *aiye* (艾 叶, Leaf of Mugwort).

Prescription: The pepper and downy *aiye* are pounded with the green onion and mixed with hot steamed rice (the hottest tolerated by the baby) for application into the umbilicus. The paste is kept in position by bandage and changed once a day.

Explanation: Chronically crying babies usually cry only at a fixed time of night, but are normal during the day.

Recipe 2: One bulb of stewed garlic and *ruxiang* (乳　香, Frankincense) 2 g.

Prescription: These ingredients are pounded to prepare pills the size of mustard seeds for an oral administration of 7 pills with milk.

Explanation: This pill is used to treat night crying of young babies due to cold in the spleen.

25. Inflammation of Umbilicus in Newborn Babies

Recipe: Green onion stalks 3 g, and fresh persimmon tree leaves 5 g.

Prescription: The ingredients are pounded to prepare a paste for application over the lesion twice a day.

Explanation: This is an infection of the umbilicus of newborn babies due to poor local hygiene. This method cannot be used for babies with fever and other general symptoms, because they need more effective treatment.

26. Umbilical Tetanus in Infants

Recipe: One handful of green onion stalks and 7 grains of white pepper.

Prescription: A powder of these ingredients is fried to make a hot cake for application on the umbilicus.

Explanation: This method is used to treat persistently crying newborn babies with protruding umbilicus and pale lips.

Chapter 6
DERMATOLOGICAL DISEASES

1. Alopecia

Recipe 1: An adequate amount of ripe ginger.

Prescription: The ginger is cut to expose a new surface with some oozing juice used to rub the bare scalp until the ginger juice dries. Then the ginger is cut again to obtain another new surface for rubbing the affected area. The same procedure may be repeated 2-3 times, and the treatment may be applied 2-3 times a day. About one week later, some fine and yellow hair may appear and then gradually turn dark and shiny.

Explanation: This method is used to treat alopecia caused by scalp infection. At the same time, the patient should pay attention to improving their nutrition.

Recipe 2: Several slices of ripe ginger and an adequate amount of Chinese sorghum liquor.

Prescription: Ginger slices are soaked in sorghum liquor for 2-3 days and then used to rub the alopecia area. The hair may regenerate half a month later.

Explanation: This method can be used to treat ordinary alopecia.

Recipe 3: Baked fresh ginger skin 30 g, and ginseng 30 g.

Prescription: A powder of these herbs is scattered over the alopecia area and rubbed with fresh ginger, once every 2 days.

Explanation: This method is more effective for treating alopecia areata.

2. Alopecia Areata

Recipe: An adequate amount of fresh ginger.

Prescription: The slices of fresh ginger are used to gently rub the alopecia area until the scalp turns flushed, 2-3 times a day.

Explanation: This method is used as a supplemental treatment together with oral administration of *guipi wan* (spleen-invigorating and heart nourishing pills) and *shiquan dabu wan* (pills of ten powerful tonics).

3. Grey Hair

Recipe: An adequate amount of garlic and ginger.

Prescription: The garlic and ginger are ground to prepare a paste for application over the scalp by rubbing. After the paste is washed away, some perfume may be applied to remove the foul odor of garlic. The paste is best applied before going to bed, once every 3 days.

Explanation: The garlic and ginger can promote metabolism. The hair may turn black 3-4 months after the application of this paste.

4. Dandruff

Recipe 1: An adequate amount of garlic.

Prescription: The garlic is pounded to squeeze juice for application on the scalp before going to bed, and water with perfume is used to wash the hair next morning for removing the foul odor of garlic. This treatment may be repeated several times.

Explanation: This garlic juice can promote blood circulation and relieve dryness of scalp to reduce the formation of dandruff.

Recipe 2: An adequate amount of green onion and Chinese chives.

Prescription: The two vegetables are washed and cut into short segments for cooking a dish by frying in oil. The dish is then eaten with bread or rice.

Explanation: This dish can relieve itching of scalp and reduce dandruff.

5. Folliculitis

Recipe: An adequate amount of green onion stalks and sesame oil.

Prescription: The sesame oil is boiled for a while and then cooled down for use. After dipping in sesame oil, the green onion stalk is used to rub the affected area for 20-30 minutes for 3 successive days.

Explanation: This method can relieve toxicity, clear heat, and resolve swelling in treating folliculitis.

6. Eyebrow Defect

Recipe: One big lump of fresh ginger, mustard seeds 15 g, and raw *banxia* (半 夏 , Ternate Pinellia) 5 g.

Prescription: A powder of mustard seeds and *banxia* is mixed with ginger juice for application with a new pen brush over the eyebrows 2 times during the day and once at night for 4-5 successive days. The eyebrows may then gradually regenerate.

Explanation: This method is also useful for congenital absence of eyebrows.

7. Acne Rosacea (Brandy Nose)

Recipe: One lump of fresh ginger, 7 pieces of *caowu* (草 乌 , Wild Aconite Root) and a small amount of musk.

Prescription: A powder of *caowu* and musk is mixed in chaulmoogra oil in a porcelain container and heated over fire. The nose is rubbed with fresh ginger first and then with this oily preparation, for 3 days.

Explanation: This method may produce a good therapeutic effect in treating brandy nose, especially in the early stages.

8. Tinea (Ringworm)

Recipe 1: An adequate amount of garlic and vaseline.

Prescription: A garlic paste is mixed with vaseline for application over the skin lesion, twice a day.

Explanation: This method can be used to treat various kinds of tinea and is especially useful in treating tinea corporis.

Recipe 2: Garlic 30 g and fresh Chinese chives 30 g.

Prescription: These ingredients are pounded to prepare a paste for application over the skin lesion.

Explanation: This method can be used to treat various tinea, including fungal infections of the skin, hair, and nails of the fingers and toes.

Recipe 3: An adequate amount of green onion, chicken eggs and Chinese prickly ash.

Prescription: These ingredients are fried in sesame oil and pounded to prepare cakes for application while still warm over the skin lesion.

Explanation: This method is used to treat stubborn tinea.

Recipe 4: An adequate amount of garlic cloves and a rusty iron utensil.

Prescription: After the iron utensil is washed clean, its rusty surface is rubbed with a garlic clove. The garlic stained with iron rust is used to rub the skin surrounding the tinea lesion until a sensation of pain and heat is detected by the patient, 3 times a day for 2 days.

Explanation: The iron rust should not be completely cleaned away when the iron utensil is washed before treatment.

Recipe 5: An adequate amount of garlic and sesame oil.

Prescription: The peeled garlic is pounded and mixed with sesame oil to prepare a paste for application over the skin lesion, once a day.

Explanation: This method is used to treat tinea of the scalp. The local burning pain sensation over the lesion after application of this paste is a normal reaction.

Recipe 6: Garlic.

Prescription: A garlic paste is mixed with sesame oil or vaseline to prepare an ointment for application over the scalp after the hair is totally cut away, once a day or every 2 days. The patient may have a burning pain sensation where the ointment has been applied.

Explanation: This preparation can kill bacteria and worms to treat tinea of the scalp, including white ringworm and yellow ringworm.

9. Psoriasis

Recipe: Garlic 50 g, and Chinese chives 50 g.

Prescription: These vegetables are pounded and warmed over fire for application over the lesion by hard rubbing, 1-2 times a day for several successive days.

Explanation: This method can relieve stagnant blood and toxicity in treating psoriasis and allergic dermatitis.

10. Dermatitis

Recipe 1: Green onion stalks 30 g, garlic with purple skin 30 g, borneol 2 g, cane sugar 30 g, and castor bean 20 g.

Prescription: After the green onion and garlic are slightly baked, the two herbs are pounded together to prepare a paste for application over the skin affected area and bound with a bandage, once a day.

Explanation: This method is used to treat neurodermatitis.

Recipe 2: Garlic 30 g, and Realgar 150 g.

Prescription: These ingredients are pounded to prepare a paste for application over the lesion, once a day.

Explanation: This method is used to treat paddy field dermatitis of the damp-heat type with local swelling and erosion.

Recipe 3: An adequate amount of garlic cloves and rice vinegar.

Prescription: The garlic is washed and pounded and the

garlic paste is wrapped in a piece of gauze and soaked in the vinegar for 2-3 hours. Then the bag of garlic paste is used to rub the lesion for 10-20 minutes, twice a day.

Explanation: This method can relieve stagnant blood and toxicity and kill worms in treating neurodermatitis.

11. Cutaneous Pruritus

Recipe: Three pieces of ripe green onion with roots and seeds.

Prescription: A hot decoction of green onion is used to wash the itching skin.

Explanation: Cutaneous pruritus is a skin disease with general itching all over the body, worse at night, and difficult to control. The patient repeatedly and forcibly scratches the itching skin until blood is drawn and pain ensues. The attack of itching may last for several minutes or several hours.

12. Urticaria

Recipe: Ginger 50 g, half a bowl of vinegar, and brown sugar 100 g.

Prescription: The shredded ginger is boiled with vinegar and sugar for about 10 minutes. After removing the dregs, a small cup of decoction is drunk after mixing with warm water, 2-3 times a day.

Explanation: This recipe can relieve stagnant blood and toxicity in treating urticaria with intractable itching caused by an allergy to fish and crab.

13. Eczema

Recipe: Three green onion stalks, *tudahuang* (土 大 黄, Rhubard) 10 g, and *sharen* (砂 仁 , Grains of Paradise) 10 g.

Prescription: A decoction of these herbs is used to wash the lesion.

Explanation: Eczema is an allergic and inflammatory skin

disease which can be classified as acute, subacute, or chronic types. Skin affected areas may appear over a limited area or all over the body in patients of any age or sex. This method can be used in treating eczema of any type.

14. Vitiligo

Recipe: An adequate amount of fresh ginger and sulfur.

Prescription: Ginger with sulfur powder is used to rub the lesion.

Explanation: This method can kill worms and relieve toxicity in treating vitiligo.

15. Tinea Versicolor

Recipe: Fresh ginger 20 g, and rice vinegar 100 ml.

Prescription: The pounded ginger is soaked in vinegar for 12 hours and stored in a closed container for use. After the lesion is washed with soap, the vinegar extract of ginger is applied over the lesion with cotton once a day, for 3 successive days.

Explanation: At the early stages of tinea versicolor, the skin lesion contains round macules, light yellow or yellowish brown in color, like a soybean in size and covered with fine furfurous scales. The small macules may fuse together to form a patch and the surrounding skin becomes paler in color than normal skin. In general, the patient has no symptoms or only some mild itching.

16. Skin Scar

Recipe: An adequate amount of ginger juice and calomel.

Prescription: These ingredients are mixed to prepare a paste for application over the lesion.

Explanation: This method is used to treat new scars of the face.

17. Herpes Zoster

Recipe 1: Two bulbs of single-clove garlic and realgar powder 10 g.

Prescription: The ingredients are pounded to prepare a paste for application over the lesion.

Explanation: The skin affected areas of this disease are clusters of vesicles, usually appearing around the trunk of the body and causing burning pain.

Recipe 2: An adequate amount of ginger.

Prescription: Ginger juice is boiled in a copper container for application over the skin lesion to produce a hot and stimulating sensation, 1-2 times a day.

Explanation: The patient may acquire lifelong immunity from this disease.

Recipe 3: An adequate amount of single-clove garlic.

Prescription: The garlic is pounded for application over the skin lesion.

Explanation: The garlic paste should not be applied over the ruptured blisters. Ordinary garlic may also be used, if no single-clove garlic is available.

18. Progressive Keratosis of Fingers and Palm

Recipe: An adequate amount of garlic.

Prescription: The garlic with stem and skin is boiled in water and the hands are put into the warm garlic decoction for 10 minutes, once each night for one month until the skin lesion heals.

Explanation: This disease is also called progressive dry sclerosis of the palm and soles.

19. Desquamation of Palm

Recipe 1: Green onion roots of 100 g, willow tree twigs 100 g, and Chinese prickly ash 100 g.

Prescription: The ingredients are boiled in 500 ml of water

on a low flame for more than 10 minutes and the warm decoction is used to wash the hands until the decoction cools.

Explanation: The skin lesion of the palm may heal after this treatment is continued for one week.

Recipe 2: An adequate amount of garlic.

Prescription: The garlic paste is applied over the palms twice a day, in the morning and at night.

Explanation: The skin lesion may heal after treatment is continued for 5 days.

20. Chilblains

Recipe 1: An adequate amount of garlic with purple skin.

Prescription: Before winter, the garlic paste is often applied over the area of old frostbite, once a day for 5-7 days. The application of garlic paste should be stopped if blisters appear.

Explanation: This method is used to prevent the recurrence of chilblains.

Recipe 2: Fresh ginger 25 g, one white radish, *baifuzi* (白附子 , Giant Typhonium) 5 g, and *guizhi* (桂 枝 , Cinnamon Twig) 25 g.

Prescription: These herbs are boiled in water and the hot decoction is used to wash the lesion twice a day. Two days' treatment may produce a therapeutic effect.

Explanation: This method is used to treat chilblains before ulceration.

Recipe 3: Fresh ginger.

Prescription: The ginger juice is boiled to prepare a paste for application to the lesion.

Explanation: This method can be used in treating chilblains of the hand and foot. The juice of fresh ginger can be used for gargling and treating aphtha in the oral cavity.

Recipe 4: Three bulbs of garlic.

Prescription: The garlic is pounded and the garlic juice is used to rub the lesion.

Explanation: The garlic juice is used to rub the area of old chilblains each morning for one week to prevent the recurrence of chilblains.

Recipe 5: Fresh ginger 25 g.

Prescription: The ginger is boiled in water and the warm ginger decoction is used to wash and rub the area of old chilblains, twice a day for 7 days.

Explanation: This method can be used in all four seasons to prevent the recurrence of chilblains.

Recipe 6: An adequate amount of garlic.

Prescription: The garlic slices are applied over the lesion for 30 minutes, twice a day.

Explanation: After the chilblains is cured by this method, it will not recur the next year.

Recipe 7: One lump of fresh ginger.

Prescription: After baking, the hot ginger is used to rub the lesion.

Explanation: This is a useful method for treating chilblains, but it cannot be used to treat ulcerated lesions.

21. Wart

Recipe: An adequate amount of fresh ginger and vinegar.

Prescription: The ginger juice is mixed with vinegar for application to the lesion.

Explanation: This method is used to treat common warts.

22. Underarm Odor

Recipe: An adequate amount of fresh ginger and tincture of iodine.

Prescription: After washing with hot water, the armpit is rubbed with fresh ginger until the local skin is flushed. The tincture of iodine is then applied over the armpit twice a day, for 15 days.

Explanation: The armpit skin should not be injured by

rubbing with ginger.

23. Clavus (Corns)

Recipe 1: One bulb of garlic with purple skin and one green onion stalks.

Prescription: The garlic and green onion are pounded and mixed with vinegar to prepare a paste. The rough layers of skin over the corn is peeled away until some blood oozes. The foot is then soaked in salt water (salt 5 g in 2,000 ml of warm boiled water) for 20 minutes to soften the skin. After the foot is dried with a towel, the garlic and green onion paste is applied over the corn and bound up with gauze, a bandage, and adhesive plaster. The paste is changed once a day or every two days for 5-7 days.

Explanation: The paste should be prepared with fresh garlic and green onion and the treatment should be continued until the corn sloughs off.

Recipe 2: An adequate amount of fresh ginger slices and *aiye* (艾　叶, Leaf of Mugwort).

Prescription: A ginger slice is put on the corn and the burned downy *aiye* is put on ginger slice. The corn may slough off two days later.

Explanation: The treatment may be repeated, if the first attempt fails.

Recipe 3: An adequate amount of garlic.

Prescription: The garlic is cut into slices of 1-2 cm in width, and a small hole is made at the center of the garlic slice to expose the corn when the garlic slice is put over it. The burned downy *aiye* is then put on the ginger slice for applying moxibustion twice a day, until the corn sloughs off.

Explanation: The moxibustion should not be very hot, otherwise it may cause a burn injury to the underlying skin.

Recipe 4: One piece of fresh green onion.

Prescription: After the foot is washed with hot water, the

white thin scale of the lower end of the green onion is put on the corn and kept in position by a piece of adhesive plaster. One day later, the tenderness of the corn may be reduced or relieved. After repeated treatment from the second day, the surrounding skin may turn white and soft and the corn may spontaneously slough off.

Explanation: This method used of treating corns does not produce any harmful effects.

Recipe 5: One green onion stalk and one water chestnut.

Prescription: The peeled green onion and water chestnut are pounded to prepare a paste for application over the corn, and bound with a bandage. The paste is changed every night before going to bed.

Explanation: This method can promote the spontaneous sloughing of corns.

Recipe 6: Fluid from green onion leaves.

Prescription: After the green onion leaves are cut from the stalk, the fluid may be squeezed from the leaves and applied to the corn several times for treatment.

Explanation: This method can soften the skin and cause spontaneous sloughing of corns after application of the fluid over for a long period of time.

24. Tinea Pedis (Tinea of Foot)

Recipe 1: An adequate amount of garlic.

Prescription: The garlic juice is applied to the lesion after the foot is washed clean.

Explanation: In patients with tender skin, the garlic juice may be diluted with water to prevent burn injuries to the skin.

Recipe 2: Twenty to twenty five cloves of peeled garlic, and vinegar 150-200 ml.

Prescription: The pounded garlic is soaked in vinegar for 2-3 days. After immersing in warm water for 3-5 minutes, the foot is put in vinegar extract of garlic for 15-20 minutes, 3 times a day for 10-15 days.

Explanation: This method is used to treat infected and ruptured lesions.

25. Eczema of Scrotum

Recipe 1: Fresh green onion stalks 90 g, and *ruxiang* powder (乳 香 , Frankincense) 3 g.

Prescription: The *ruxiang* powder is mixed with green onion juice for application over the affected area, 2-3 times a day.

Explanation: According to the theory of traditional Chinese medicine, this disease is caused by stagnation of wind, and dampness and heat pathogens in the skin and muscles.

Recipe 2: One slice of fresh ginger and *shihu* (石 斛 , Dendrobium) 6 g.

Prescription: These herbs are boiled to prepare a tea for repeated drinking.

Explanation: This method can be used in combination with other recipes to treat eczema of the scrotum.

26. Impetigo

Recipe: An adequate amount of green onion with roots.

Prescription: The green onion is pounded and mixed with honey for application over the lesion.

Explanation: Impetigo is a pyogenic skin disease infected by direct contact, and usually appears over the head, face, hands, arms, and legs. It is more common in children. This method is effective for treating impetigo.

27. Chronic Ulceration in Perineal Region

Recipe: An adequate amount of green onion stalks, yellow wine, and sesame oil.

Prescription: After sundrying, the green onion stalks are fried while yellow wine is continuously sprayed over them until they turn yellow in color. The fried green onion is then ground and mixed with sesame oil to prepare a paste for application to the lesion.

Explanation: This method is used to treat chronic perineal ulceration.

Chapter 7
DISEASES OF EAR, NOSE AND THROAT

1. Rhinitis

Recipe 1: An adequate amount of garlic and glycerine twice the weight of the garlic.

Prescription: The garlic is pounded to squeeze juice and mixed with glycerine for application into nostrils with cotton balls after the nose is washed with normal saline.

Explanation: Honey may be used instead of glycerine.

Recipe 2: An adequate amount of green onion stalks.

Prescription: After the nasal cavity is washed with normal saline at night, the green onion stalks are pounded to squeeze juice for application with cotton balls into both nostrils alternately to avoid interfering with breath.

Explanation: Green onion stalks are useful for treating rhinitis and nasal sinusitis.

Recipe 3: Five slices of fresh ginger and green onion stalk 5 g.

Prescription: Buckwheat flour is mixed with a decoction of the above ingredients to prepare small cakes for application at Hegu (LI 4) acupoint, and then it is removed after it has dried.

Explanation: The Hegu acupoint lies on the dorsum of the hand between the first and second metacarpal bones. This method can also be used to treat nasal obstruction in children.

Recipe 4: One bulb of garlic.

Prescription: The garlic juice is diluted by a twofold amount of boiled water for nose drops.

Explanation: The garlic juice can clear heat accumulated in the lungs to resolve local inflammation.

2. Nasal Bleeding

Recipe 1: Garlic 12 g, fresh ginger 2 g, *aiye* (艾 叶 , Leaf of Mugwort) 12 g, and one egg white.

Prescription: The ingredients are pounded and applied over the soles of the feet.

Explanation: This method is used to treat nasal bleeding due to deficiency of spleen qi and failure to adjust normal blood circulation.

Recipe 2: Two or three cloves of fresh garlic.

Prescription: The garlic paste is spread to the size of a çoin over a piece of cloth and applied to the sole on the side opposite from the bleeding nostril until pain or a blister appears on the sole (applied to both soles, if bleeding from both nostrils).

Explanation: This method is useful for stopping nosebleed of any reason, especially effective in nasal bleeding caused by inflammation of the nasal cavity.

3. Toothache

Recipe 1: One green onion stalk and alum 15 g.

Prescription: A paste of these ingredients is applied to the painful tooth and changed every 5 hours.

Explanation: Toothache is a symptom of many diseases of the teeth or periodontitis. This method can be used to treat toothache due to many causes, such as excessive fire, deficient fire, or caries.

Recipe 2: Two cloves of large ripe garlic and calomelas 5 g.

Prescription: These herbs are pounded and applied on the Jingqu (LU 8) acupoint and covered with a small clam shell or other substance. The paste is removed when an irriting sensation is detected and a blister appears underneath the paste. The pain may be relieved after the blister is punctured and the yellow fluid inside the blister is discharged.

Explanation: The Jingqu acupoint is located at the proximal end of thumb and in a small depression between styloid process of radius and radial artery.

Recipe 3: Fresh ginger 6 g, garlic 6 g, tea leaves 12 g, and *weilingxian* (威 灵 仙 , Clematis Root) 12 g.

Prescription: These herbs are pounded and mixed with sesame oil and egg white to prepare a paste for application at Hegu (LI 4) and Yongquan (KI 1) acupoints.

Explanation: This method is used to treat toothache due to deficiency of kidney yin and the flaming up of deficient fire.

Recipe 4: Two or three bulbs of single-clove garlic.

Prescription: The peeled garlic is baked over a stove and the hot garlic clove is cut open for application on the painful area. The garlic may be changed several times after it cools down.

Explanation: This method can kill bacteria and relieve toxicity in treating toothache.

Recipe 5: Fresh ginger 100 g and towel gourd 500 g.

Prescription: The fresh towel gourd is cut into cubes and the fresh ginger is cut into slices and they are boiled in water over 3 hours for oral administration, twice a day.

Explanation: This method can clear heat, relieve toxicity, resolve swelling and stop pain to treat swelling and pain of gum, dryness of mouth and nose and nasal bleeding.

4. Periodontitis

Recipe: Dried ginger 6 g, charred red date (with therapeutic effect preserved) 6 g, and dried alum 6 g.

Prescription: A powder of these herbs is applied over the lesion.

Explanation: This method is used to treat periodontitis, a common chronic disease of tissues around the tooth, more common in middle-aged and old patients.

5. Aphtha of Mouth Cavity

Recipe 1: Baked ginger 9 g, 3 pieces of *mubiezi* (木 鳖 子, Cochinchina Momordicae) and *wuzhuyu* (吴 茱 萸, Evodia Fruit) 9 g.

Prescription: A powder of these herbs is mixed with water for application to the umbilicus which is then covered with a piece of paper.

Explanation: Aphtha of the mouth is characterized by yellowish white ulcers the size of a soybean on the oral mucosa. It is divided into excessive and deficient types.

Recipe 2: Dried ginger (baked to a dark color) 9 g and *huanglian* (黄 连, Goldthread) 15 g.

Prescription: A powder of these herbs is applied over the affected areas, which may heal after excretion of saliva is induced.

Explanation: This method may produce a good effect in treating ulceration of the mouth cavity and tongue with difficulty swallowing.

6. Sore Throat

Recipe 1: Two bulbs of garlic.

Prescription: The garlic paste is applied at Yuji (LU 10) and Dazhui (GV 14) acupoints.

Explanation: This method can clear heat in the lungs to treat swelling and throat pain due to an attack by ascending lung heat.

Recipe 2: Small single-clove garlic 30 g, and vinegar 50 ml.

Prescription: The garlic is pounded in vinegar for application over the affected area.

Explanation: This method can resolve swelling and control pain in treating sore throat due to an upward attack of wind, cold, dampness, and heat pathogens.

Recipe 3: One lump of ripe ginger and a handful of *cangerzi* (苍 耳 子, Cocklebur Fruit).

Prescription: After grinding the herbs, the juice obtained by squeezing is mixed with a small spoonful of liquor for one oral administration.

Explanation: Fresh ginger with a pungent taste can expel pathogen from the body surface and *cangerzi* can clear heat and relieve toxicity in treating swelling and sore throat.

Recipe 4: Equal amounts of dried ginger and *banxia* (半 夏, Ternate Pinellia), washed with boiled water.

Prescription: A small amount of powder of these herbs is applied to the tongue and throat.

Explanation: This method can be used to treat sore throat with fever and other throat diseases.

7. Laryngitis

Recipe 1: One bulb of single-clove garlic.

Prescription: The garlic paste is applied at Yangxi (LI 5) acupoint and then removed after a blister is formed.

Explanation: The blister should be protected from rupture and infection. The Yangxi acupoint is proximal to the Hegu (LI 4) acupoint and lies in a depression as the thumb is tilted.

Recipe 2: Fresh ginger juice 5 ml and white radish juice 5 ml.

Prescription: The two juices are mixed for oral administration with water.

Explanation: This recipe can be used to treat both acute and chronic laryngitis, but is more effective for chronic laryngitis.

8. Diphtheria

Recipe: One slice of ripe garlic.

Prescription: The garlic paste is applied at Jingqu (LU 8) acupoint until a blister is formed and punctured to empty the fluid. The Jingqu acupoint lies at the proximal end of the thumb and in a small depression between styloid process of radius and radial artery.

Explanation: The garlic can produce a therapeutic effect in treating diphtheria.

9. Aphonia

Recipe 1: An adequate amount of ginger and radish.

Prescription: The two vegetables are squeezed to prepare a juice for oral administration.

Explanation: The radish can promote discharge of gas and relieve stagnation of food, and the ginger can expel pathogens. The combined use of radish and ginger can treat aphonia due to the reduction of vital activity.

Recipe 2: An adequate amount of fresh ginger.

Prescription: The ginger is pounded to squeeze juice for repeated drinking.

Explanation: This method is used to treat sudden aphonia due to emotional disturbance or an attack of external pathogen.

10. Hoarseness of Voice

Recipe 1: Two cloves of garlic.

Prescription: The garlic paste is applied at Jingqu (LU 8) acupoint and covered with a small clam shell or other substance. An irritating sensation then will be detected and a blister will appear under the garlic paste. The blister is then punctured with a needle to empty the yellow fluid.

Explanation: This method is useful for treating hoarseness of the voice caused by pharyngitis and laryngitis.

Recipe 2: Garlic 6 g, fresh ginger 3 g, *aiye* (艾 叶, Leaf of Mugwort) 20 g, and one egg white.

Prescription: These ingredients are pounded for application at the Dazhui (GV 14) and Yongquan (KI 1) acupoints.

Explanation: This method can be used to treat hoarseness caused by wind-heat or wind-cold pathogen.

11. Foreign Body in Throat

Recipe 1: An adequate amount of fresh ginger and chicken blood.

Prescription: The ginger is squeezed to produce juice for oral administration after mixing with chicken blood.

Explanation: This method is used to treat the adhesion of sticky food or other substances in the throat.

Recipe 2: One clove of garlic and some sugar.

Prescription: The garlic clove is horizontally cut into two pieces and separately inserted into each nostril to block the breath. At the same time, a spoonful of sugar is swallowed without water. This treatment can be repeated.

Explanation: This method is used to dislodge fish bones stuck in the throat.

Recipe 3: One bulb of single-clove garlic.

Prescription: The garlic is inserted into the nostrils.

Explanation: This method is used to treat fish bones lodged in the throat.

12. Conjunctivitis

Recipe 1: One piece of fresh ginger and *huanglian* (黄 连 , Goldthread)) 1.5 g.

Prescription: After a small hole is made in the ginger and *huanglian* is placed into the hole, it is baked over fire for application of the hot ginger with *huanglian* on the Taiyang (EX-HN 5) acupoint.

Explanation: Conjunctivitis is an acute infectious disease of eye with a tendency to progress violently. It is usually caused by an attack of external wind-heat pathogen.

Recipe 2: An adequate amount of fresh ginger.

Prescription: The ginger slices are applied around the infected eye.

Explanation: This method is used to treat fire eye and red eye with infection, swelling, and pain due to other causes.

13. Itching of Eye

Recipe 1: One lump of dried ginger.

Prescription: The dried ginger is cut into a smooth, round end for applying pressure to the depression of the inner canthus until some juice is produced. It is applied again at the inner canthus after the juice is removed.

Explanation: This method is used to treat itching and eye pain.

Recipe 2: An adequate amount of ginger powder, dried alum, and borex.

Prescription: A powder of these herbs is mixed with saliva to prepare small pills the size of millet for application on the inner canthus.

Explanation: This pill can produce a good therapeutic effect in controlling intractable itching of the eye.

14. Profuse Lacrimation

Recipe: Dried ginger powder 15 g, realgar powder 30 g and *xixin* (细 辛, Wildginger) 30 g.

Prescription: The finest powder, obtained by straining the rough powder of these ingredients in a very fine sieve, is applied in a small amount into the eye, which is then washed with normal saline the next morning, for 10 successive days.

Explanation: This method is used to treat blurred vision and profuse lacrimation caused by blowing wind.

15. Deafness

Recipe 1: Two drops of green onion juice.

Prescription: Green onion juice is dropped into the ear meatus.

Explanation: Green onion juice can remove stagnant blood and open sense organ orifices to treat deafness due to external trauma with stagnant blood.

Recipe 2: Green onion juice 3 g, ginger juice 1 g, *jinpencao*

(金 盆 草) 20 g, and *shichangpu* (石 菖 蒲 , Rock Sweetflag)
20 g.

Prescription: These herbs are pounded to prepare a juice for
application into the ear.

Explanation: This method is used to treat deafness and
tinnitus due to external trauma or deficiency of kidney essence,
weakness of the spleen and stomach.

Recipe 3: One clove of garlic and one piece of croton.

Prescription: The peeled croton is baked on a low flame and
put into a hole made in the garlic clove and is then wrapped
with new cotton and put into the ear, 3-4 times to obtain a
therapeutic effect.

Explanation: This method is used to treat deafness over a
long period of time.

16. Otitis Media

Recipe: One clove of garlic and distilled water 10 ml.

Prescription: The garlic juice obtained by pounding the
garlic is mixed with distilled water for an application of several
drops into the ear, several times in a day.

Explanation: This method is used to treat otitis media,
especially useful for pyogenic infection of the middle ear.

17. Insect in Ear

Recipe 1: An adequate amount of green onion juice and
sesame oil.

Prescription: The insect may spontaneously come out of the
ear after dropping this fluid into the ear.

Explanation: This is a useful folk treatment to drive an
insect out of the ear. If it fails, the patient should visit an ENT
specialist to remove the insect.

Recipe 2: An adequate amount of green onion juice.

Prescription: The green onion juice is applied into the ear to
drive the insect out.

Explanation: After the insect out, the ear meatus should be cleaned by irrigation.

图书在版编目(CIP)数据

葱姜蒜治百病:英文/王富春,段育华主编. —北京:外文出版社,1998
(中国传统医疗实用小丛书)
ISBN 7 - 119 - 01905 - 8

Ⅰ.葱… Ⅱ.①王… ②段… Ⅲ.①葱 - 中草药 - 临床应用 - 英文 ②姜 - 中
草药 - 临床应用 - 英文 ③蒜 - 中草药 - 临床应用 - 英文 Ⅳ.R282.710.7

中国版本图书馆 CIP 数据核字 (97) 第 05011 号

责任编辑　郭保芹
封面设计　王　志

外文出版社网址:

　http://www.flp.com.cn

外文出版社电子信箱:

　info@flp.com.cn

　sales@flp.com.cn

葱姜蒜治百病

王富春　段育华　主编

*

©外文出版社
外文出版社出版
(中国北京百万庄大街 24 号)
邮政编码 100037
北京外文印刷厂印刷
中国国际图书贸易总公司发行
(中国北京车公庄西路 35 号)
北京邮政信箱第 399 号　邮政编码 100044
1998 年(大 32 开)第 1 版
2000 年第 1 版第 2 次印刷
(英)
ISBN 7 - 119 - 01905 - 8/R·140(外)
03480
14 - E - 3120P